PATHOPHYSIOLOGY
Concepts of Altered Health States

FOURTH EDITION

Carol Mattson Porth
R.N., M.S.N., Ph.D. (Physiology)

Professor, School of Nursing
University of Wisconsin - Milwaukee

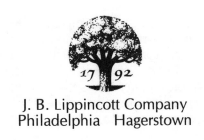

J. B. Lippincott Company
Philadelphia   Hagerstown

Sponsoring Editor: Diana Schweisguth

Sponsoring Editorial Assistant: Sarah L. Andrus

Ancillary Coordinator: Doris S. Wray

Printer/Binder: Capitol City Press

Desktop Compositor: Richard G. Hartley

7   6   5   4   3   2

0-397-55126-6

PATHOPHYSIOLOGY

Concepts of Altered Health States

Introduction

The purpose of this instructor's manual is to assist faculty in using the textbook *Pathophysiology: Concepts of Altered Health States* in their teaching assignments. The manual is organized into two sections. The first section follows the unit organization of the book and contains suggested teaching-learning strategies including glossary terms and test items. The second section contains a set of transparency masters.

About the Textbook

Pathophysiology: Concepts of Altered Health was written with the intent of serving as both a textbook and as a reference source. Instructors may want to keep this in mind as they make assignments from the book.

The book was designed to facilitate learning. There are learning objectives at the beginning of each chapter. Each major section of a chapter begins with an introductory paragraph and ends with a summary paragraph. Most students are visual learners; therefore, carefully selected figures have been included throughout the book. Tables and charts, designed to emphasize important content, have also been included. Most chapters contain bibliography references. These references have been selected because of their relevance, comprehensive nature, and area of understanding.

The content of the book has been organized into three areas of focus: (1) control of normal function, (2) altered function or pathophysiology, and (3) when appropriate, system or organ failure. For some students the chapters or sections that deal with normal anatomy and physiology will be a review and for others the content will represent new learning. Assignments can be made accordingly.

Pathophysiology: Concepts of Altered Health uses a conceptual model that integrates alterations in health across the life cycle. Chapters 6 and 7 focus on the developmental aspects of altered health in children and older adults. These chapters were designed to serve as a conceptual model for understanding integrated content on children and older adults that is presented in other sections of the book. The book also integrates physiologic mechanisms of drug therapy and other treatment modalities. This content was not intended to replace a pharmacology or other nursing texts, but to help the student form relationships and provide the rationale for various treatment modalities, their possible interactions, and potential adverse effects.

About teaching pathophysiology

The teaching of a course in pathophysiology can be an exciting and rewarding experience. Pathophysiology, or as this author would prefer, the physiology of altered health states, is a dynamic science that has application for both well and sickly populations of all age groups. It is the magnificence of the human body as it continuously monitors and adjusts to the stresses of everyday life, albeit in health or disease that make a course in pathophysiology interesting to instructors and students alike. Most importantly, each student brings to the course their own physiological functioning against which they can compare what occurs in states of altered health.

Using an altered health framework allows the instructor to focus on the physiologic responses to altered health states rather than the pathology of the disease process itself. It also prepares and motivates the student to consider the social and psychological implications of human responses such as anxiety, pain, breathlessness, and fatigue and thereby facilitates the development and use of nursing diagnoses. For the most part the book focuses on common health problems rather than rare disease states. For example, full chapters have been devoted to hypertension and diabetes mellitus.

Regardless of how your curriculum is structured, there is seldom time to cover all of the topics addressed in the book. If your class time is limited you will have to decide (1) what topics to cover, (2) what sequence to present them in, and (3) how much time to assign to each unit. Instructors may want to consider sequencing the course content so that foundational concepts such as neoplasia and alterations in fluids and electrolytes are covered at the beginning of the course and then reinforced in subsequent classes rather than repeated.

Students often become overwhelmed with large reading assignments. It is suggested that assignments be tailored to meet the objectives of the course. In some situations, it may be desirable to assign selected pages rather than an entire chapter.

About the Instructors Manual

The instructors manual includes suggestions for selected classroom teaching strategies and student learning activities. There is a description of transparency masters included at the end of the manual and suggestions for their use; other teaching strategies and demonstrations; and selected student learning experiences and activities. One of these learning activities is the development of a student glossary. The author has found that many students have had minimal exposure to medical terminology and that this often impedes their understanding of pathophysiology content. Thus, one of the teaching strategies for each chapter is a list of terms for students to define and include in their glossaries. Since terms that appear in beginning chapters of the book are not repeated in subsequent chapters, instructors who do not use these chapters may want to add terms from their earlier chapters to their assignments. Instructors may also want to include commonly used prefixes, root words, and suffixes to their list of glossary terms.

The author has also found that preprinted lecture notes are useful in assisting students with notetaking. This is especially helpful for students who write slowly. Local copy centers will often duplicate the lecture notes and make them available to students at a reasonable price. The availability of preprinted lecture notes allows the student to focus on the lecture content, adding their own comments as needed. Study questions, short case studies, glossary terms, and other student learning aids can be included in the lecture note package.

Table of Contents

Alterations in Cell Function and Growth

Unit 1 provides an overview of cell structure and function, adaptive cellular responses and mechanisms of cell injury, genetic control of both inheritance and cell function, genetic and congenital disorders, and neoplasia. The chapters in this unit contain information that is necessary in order to understand the content in subsequent chapters. This unit, particularly Chapters 1 and 3, will be a review for some students; for others, this content will be new.

Chapter 1

Cell and Tissue Characteristics

Chapter 1 presents the reader with a description of the normal structure and function of body cells. It contains information on aerobic and anaerobic cell metabolism. In order to prevent repetition, this chapter contains a discussion of membrane potentials—content needed for understanding cardiac function, the effects of fluids and electrolytes on various body functions, and the nervous system. The chapter also includes a discussion of tissue types including epithelial tissue, connective tissue, and muscle tissue. The molecular mechanisms of muscle contraction are included in this chapter.

Teaching strategies

— Overhead transparencies

Figure 1-1 provides a composite view of the components of a cell.

Figure 1-6 depicts the cell membrane with its water-soluble and water-insoluble layers, the protein carrier molecules as transport vehicles, and cell surface receptor sites. It is important to emphasize that some of the protein molecules serve as cell surface antigens (HLA antigens that will be discussed in Chapter 13).

Figures 1-20 shows the arrangement of muscle fiber structures, and the relationship between actin and myosin filaments when the muscle is stretched or contracted. These figures can also be used when discussing myocardial contractility and Starling's law of the heart in Chapters 20 and 21.

—Glossary terms

anabolism	glycolysis
action potential	heterophagy
adenosine triphosphate (ATP)	hyperpolarization
	hypopolarization
autophagy	lysosome
catabolism	metabolism (aerobic and anaerobic)
chromatin	
cytoplasm	nexus
depolarization	nucleoli
desmosome	parenchymal
diffusion	phagocytosis

1

pinocytosis

protoplasm

organelles

osmosis

refractory period
(absolute and
relative)

repolarization

sarcolemma

sarcoplasm

—Other teaching strategies

A. Have students label the parts of a cell and describe their functions.

B. Have students use a calculator with log function to calculate the equilibrium potential with different serum potassium levels when the cell is permeable to potassium and impermeable to sodium, and with different serum sodium levels when the cell is permeable to sodium and impermeable to potassium.

Chapter 2

Cellular Adaptation/Injury And Wound Healing

When confronted with stresses, body cells undergo changes in size and structure that permit survival and maintenance of essential functions. Chapter 2 describes normal cellular adaptations including atrophy, hypertrophy, hyperplasia, metaplasia, and dysplasia. The chapter also includes a discussion of cell injury and tissue repair and wound healing.

Teaching strategies
—Glossary terms

atrophy

denervation

degeneration

dysplasia

enzyme

free radical

gangrene

granulation tissue

ischemia

hyperplasia

hypertrophy

metaplasia

necrosis

radiation (ionizing, ultra violet)

regeneration

vasoconstriction

—Other teaching strategies

A. Develop a list of tissue injuries (e.g. burns, freezing, etc.,) and have the students describe the mechanism of injury and types of tissue changes that would be expected.

Chapter 3

Genetic Control of Cell Function and Inheritance

Genes determine the types of proteins and enzymes that are made by the cell. Thus, they control not only inheritance, but the day-to-day function of all of the cells in the body. Chapter 3 describes the genetic control of cell structure and function, chromosomes, patterns of inheritance, genetic control of protein synthesis, regulation of gene function, and gene technology. It is recommended that this chapter be used as an introduction to Chapter 4.

Teaching strategies

—Overhead transparencies

Figure 3-7 shows the stages of cell mitosis and illustrates the importance of the mitotic spindle in the process.

> Note: Instructors may also want to prepare an overhead transparency of the genetic code (Table 3-1) to illustrate how the genetic code is used in protein synthesis.

—Glossary terms

anaphase	metaphase
autosomes	mitosis
Barr body	mosacism
clone	mutation
expressivity	nucleotide
gene	pedigree
gene loci	penetrance
gene expression	phenotype
gene repression	polygenic
genotype	prophase
heterozygous	recessive trait
homozygous	recombinant DNA technology
hybridization	
ideogram	semiconservatism
induction	transcription
karyotype	translocation
linkage	zygote

—Other teaching strategies

A. Have the students use their ABO blood type to develop a phenotype and genotype of their blood type.

Chapter 4

Genetic and Congenital Disorders

Chapter 4 provides an overview of genetic and chromosomal disorders, congenital disorders arising from in utero exposure to environmental agents, and methods used in the diagnosis of genetic and congenital disorders. The chapter is organized into three parts: (1) genetic and chromosomal disorders, (2) disorders due to environmental influences, and (3) diagnosis and counseling. The chapter also provides an overview of two current health problems related to in utero exposure to potential teratogenic agents: fetal alcohol syndrome and cocaine abuse during pregnancy.

Teaching strategies

—Glossary terms

amniocentesis	diploid
chorionic villus sampling	haploid
	meiosis
monosomy	trisomy
polymorphism	teratogenic
translocation	ultrasonography

—Other teaching strategies

A. Obtain an ultrasound picture of a fetus for students to examine. One of the students in the class may be able to supply a picture and describe the experience of having ultrasound done.

B. Have students write a short paper on a current health problem related to in utero exposure to a teratogenic agent.

Chapter 5

Alterations in Cell Differentiation: Neoplasia

Chapter 5 provides a general overview of neoplasia—a disorder of cell proliferation and differentiation. The chapter begins with a discussion of cell growth and differentiation. The discussion of cell growth and differentiation is followed by a discussion of the terminology that is used in describing neoplasms; the characteristics of benign and malignant neoplasms; the proposed role of heredity, oncogenes and oncogenic viruses, chemical carcinogens, radiation, and immunologic defects in the development of cancers; factors related to the growth and spread of tumors; and the general clinical effects of neoplasms. In addition, the chapter includes a discussion of diagnostic methods used in early detection of cancer, staging and grading of tumors, and methods of cancer treatment including surgery, radiation, and pharmacologic therapy. The chapter does not deal with specific types of cancer, but provides the basis for understanding cancers of various organs and body systems that are discussed in subsequent chapters.

Teaching strategies

—Overhead transparencies

Note: Instructors may want to prepare an additional overhead transparency that shows the determinants of cell differentiation (what a cell looks like, how it functions, and how long it lives) as a method of describing alterations in body function that occur with various types of cancers.

—Glossary terms

adjuvant	mitosis
anaplasia	mutation
aneuploidy	neoplasm
benign	oncogenes
biopsy	palliative
carcinogen	paraneoplastic syndromes
carcinoma	
cell cycle	parenchymal
cytology	phototherapy
differentiation	polyploidy
histology	proliferation
in situ	radiosensitivity
malignant	stem cell
metastasis	sarcoma

—Other teaching strategies

A. Contact the local division or district of the American Cancer Society to obtain teaching materials and information about the services of the organization such as breast and testicular self-examination and screening programs for early detection of cancer.

Examination questions

1. Which one of the following is the most abundant component of body cells:

    a. electrolytes
    • b. water
    c. proteins
    d. lipids

2. The chromatin material in the cell nucleus consists of:

    a. lysosomes
    b. ribosomes
    c. microtubules
    • d. chromosomes

3. The microsomal system for drug metabolism in the liver is contained in which one of the following cell structures:

    • a. endoplasmic reticulum
    b. ribosomes
    c. lysosomes
    d. mitochrondria

4. Which one of the following types of RNA transcribes and carries the DNA code for protein synthesis to the cytoplasm:

    • a. messenger RNA
    b. transfer RNA
    c. ribosomal RNA

5. The mitochondria function is:

    • a. transforming food constituents to cellular energy
    b. building protein molecules
    c. breaking down worn out cell parts

6. The structure of the cell membrane renders it highly permeable to:

    a. proteins
    • b. lipids
    c. electrolytes
    d. carbohydrates

7. The mechanism that moves substances across a cell membrane against a concentration gradient (from lower to higher concentration) is:

    • a. active transport
    b. diffusion
    c. osmosis
    d. phagocytosis

8. The movement of water across a semipermeable membrane in response to an uneven distribution of nondiffusible particles is called:

    a. diffusion
    b. active transport
    • c. osmosis
    d. phagocytosis

9. Osmosis is determined by:

    • a. the number of particles
    b. the size of the particles
    c. the charge of a particle
    d. the weight of a particle

10. A characteristic of epithelial tissue is that it:

- a. has no blood vessels of its own
  b. is unable to regenerate
  c. serves to connect and hold tissues together
  d. is designed for movement functions

11. Catabolism is a process in which:

- a. body tissues are broken down and used for energy
  b. food products are converted to energy sources and stored

12. A by-product of anaerobic metabolism is:

  a. adenosine triphosphate (ATP)
- b. lactic acid
  c. carbon dioxide
  d. ketoacids

13. An example of a connective tissue is:

  a. functioning cells of glandular tissue
  b. skeletal muscle fibers
  c. epidermis of the skin
- d. cartilage of a joint

14. An action potential consists of:

- a. achievement of the threshold potential, depolarization, repolarization, and re-establishment of a resting membrane potential
  b. depolarization of the membrane only
  c. membrane depolarization and repolarization
  d. achievement of threshold potential and depolarization of the membrane

15. The relative refractory period of an action potential is the time interval during which:

  a. the membrane cannot be re-excited to undergo a second action potential
- b. a stronger-than-normal stimuli can incite a second action potential

16. Hyperpolarization indicates that a nerve will require:

- a. a greater stimulus to initiate an action potential
  b. a lesser stimulus to initiate an action potential

17. Normal adaptive cell responses:

- a. occur in response to an appropriate stimuli
  b. continue once the need for the adaptive response ceases
  c. are not reversible
  d. occur in response to both appropriate and inappropriate stimuli

18. Atrophy is characterized by:

- a. a shrinkage in cell size
  b. an enlargement in cell size
  c. tissue necrosis
  d. reduction in cell numbers

19. Which one of the following types of adaptive cell responses has the potential to progress to neoplasia:

  a. atrophy
  b. hyperplasia
  c. metaplasia
- d. dysplasia

20. The term degeneration usually implies cellular injuries that are:

  a. indicative of necrosis
- b. reversible and compatible with cell survival
  c. associated with cellular accumulation of exogenous or endogenous pigments
  d. equated with cell death

21. Tissue necrosis that results from an interruption in blood flow usually results in:

- a. dry gangrene
  b. wet gangrene
  c. gas gangrene

22. The elevation of serum enzymes on laboratory tests usually implies:

    a. excessive production by cellular enzymes

    b. impaired breakdown of cellular enzymes

    • c. cell membrane injury that permits leakage of intracellular enzymes into the extracellular fluid

    d. excess production of extracellular enzymes

23. Injury due to electricity is most severe in:

    a. tissues that freely conduct electrical current

    • b. tissues that have a high resistance to flow of electrical current

24. Radiation sources such as ultrasound and microwaves exert their effects on body tissues through:

    a. breaking of chemical bonds and ionization of cell molecules

    • b. vibration and rotation of cell molecules

25. Biological agents such as bacteria and viruses differ from other injurious agents in terms of their ability to:

    a. affect tissues throughout the body

    b. cause cell death

    • c. replicate and produce continued injury

    d. produce reversible cell injury

26. Induction is a process whereby:

    • a. gene function is increased

    b. gene function is decreased

    c. gene activity is changed so that it transcribes a different message

    d. gene replication or reproduction errors occur

27. A Barr body represents the presence of:

    a. an active Y chromosome

    b. an inactive Y chromosome

    • c. an active X chromosome

    d. an inactive X chromosome

28. The phenotype refers to:

    a. all of the genetic information present in an individual's chromosomes

    b. the pattern of inheritance that was derived from either the mother or the father, but not both

    • c. the recognizable traits of an individual that are determined by his/her genes

    d. a picture of an individual's chromosomes that was constructed through genetic studies

29. A person possessing identical genes at a given locus or loci is called a:

    • a. homozygote

    b. heterozygote

30. A recessive trait is one that develops as the result of:

    • a. homozygous pairing of genes

    b. heterozygous pairing of genes

31. The best definition of a congenital disorder is one that:

    a. is due to heredity

    b. exists at birth

    • c. is caused by intrauterine exposure to a environmental agent

    d. develops after birth

32. A teratogen is:

    a. a faulty gene

    • b. an agent that causes physical defects in a developing embryo

    c. an agent that impairs meiosis

    d. a test for fetal anomalies

33. A parent that is affected with an autosomal dominant disorder has:

    a. no chance of transmitting the disorder to his/her offspring
●   b. a 25% chance of transmitting the disorder to his/her offspring
    c. a 50% chance of transmitting the disorder to his/her offspring
    d. a 50% chance of transmitting the disorder to offspring of similar sex

34. Mosacism describes:

●   a. the presence, in one individual, of 2 or more cell lines with different chromosome arrangements
    b. alterations in chromosome number
    c. alterations in chromosome structure
    d. alterations in gene structure

35. The most vulnerable period for the embryo in terms of defects arising from exposure to environmental agents is:

    a. at the time of conception
●   b. days 15 to 60 of gestation
    c. days 35 to 120 of gestation
    d. the last 3 months of gestation

36. The adverse effects of alcohol on fetal development:

    a. is limited to the first trimester of pregnancy
    b. is greatest during the second trimester of pregnancy
    c. occurs before a woman realizes she is pregnant
●   d. may exert its effects throughout pregnancy

37. In malignant neoplasia, cell proliferation:

    a. occurs in response to need
    b. ceases when the needs of the organism are met
    c. produces normally functioning cells
●   d. occurs in response to an inappropriate stimuli

38. An adenocarcinoma is:

    a. a malignant tumor of mesenchymal origin
    b. a benign tumor of mesenchymal origin
●   c. a malignant tumor of epithelial cell origin
    d. a benign tumor of epithelial cell origin

39. Cell differentiation:

    a. determines cell structure
    b. determines cell function
    c. controls cell mitosis
●   d. determines cell structure, function, and life span

40. The term anaplasia refers to:

    a. atypical cellular mitosis
●   b. lack of cell differentiation
    c. proneness to undergo necrosis
    d. uncontrolled cell growth

41. The site of cancer that has shown the greatest increases in recent years is:

    a. bone
    b. head and neck
    c. breast
●   d. lung

42. In contrast to malignant tumors, benign tumors:

●   a. are well differentiated but have lost their ability to control cell replication
    b. are more likely to undergo degenerative changes than malignant tumors
    c. do not cause pressure damage to surrounding tissues as do malignant tumors
    d. are unable to effect alterations in body function through the elaboration of hormones or other chemicals

43. One of the most important determinants of alteration in body function due to benign neoplasia is the:

   a. duration of altered cellular growth location of the neoplasia
   • b. location of the tumor
   c. agent responsible for the alteration in growth
   d. hereditary factors

44. In which one of the following types of cancer is heredity thought to play a role:

   a. lung cancer
   • b. retinoblastoma
   c. cancer of the cervix
   d. cancer of the scrotum

45. A carcinogen is an agent that is capable of inducing a mutation in:

   • a. a dividing cell line
   b. cells that fully differentiated and no longer dividing

46. Hematologic cancers differ from solid cancer tumors in terms of their:

   a. cause
   b. progress
   • c. early dissemination throughout the body
   d. differentiation

47. The rate of growth of a malignant tumor is related to:

   • a. the number of cells that are actively moving through the cell cycle during a given time and the cell cycle time
   b. the cause of the cancer and the life span of the cancer cells
   c. the age of the person that has the cancer and the number of cells that are moving through the cell cycle
   d. the location of the cancer and the cell cycle time

48. A pap smear can be done on:

   a. tissue samples
   • b. cells obtained from any body fluids or secretions
   c. only on secretions and scraping obtained from the uterine cervix
   d. serum and blood samples

49. The seven warning signals of cancer include:

   a. pain, persistent cough, a sore that doesn't heal
   b. unexplained lump in the breast or elsewhere, difficulty in swallowing, sudden shortness of breath
   • c. hoarseness, unusual bleeding or discharge, change in bowel habits
   d. fever, pain, unexplained lump in the breast or elsewhere

50. The TNM system for classifying cancers is used to describe:

   a. the microscopic nature of the cancer
   • b. the clinical spread of the disease
   c. the etiologic factors associated with the disease
   d. the location of the cancer

Developmental Aspects of Altered Health

Unit II is designed to provide an overview of developmental changes that occur during childhood and older adulthood and relate these changes to common health problems of these two age groups. This unit is intended as an introduction for specific health problems of children and the elderly that appear in other chapters of the text.

Chapter 6

Concepts of Altered Health in Children

Chapter 6 provides the reader description of normal developmental changes that occur during: (1) prenatal growth, (2) infancy, (3) early childhood, (4) the early school years to late childhood, and (5) adolescence. The chapter also includes content on the common health problems of these age groups.

Teaching Strategies

— Glossary terms

Apgar score

brachial plexus

caput succedaneum

cephalocaudal

cephalohematoma

embryo

fetus

intraventricular hemorrhage

large for gestational age

macrosomia

mean, standard deviation, median, and percentiles

necrotizing endocolitis

premature infant

proportional and disproportional growth

proximodistal

respiratory distress syndrome

small for gestational age

zygote

— Other teaching strategies

Prepare case studies with infant weight and charactertics and have students estimate gestational age using the weight graph on page 108 and the Dubowitz method on page 110.

Chapter 7

Concepts of Altered Health in Older Adults

Chapter 7 focuses on biopsychosocial changes that occur with aging and their impact on health problems of the elderly. The chapter is organized into five sections that describe: (1) who are the elderly, (2) theories of aging, (3) physical changes that occur with aging, (4) functional problems of aging, and (5) drug therapy in older adults. Instructors will want to emphasize that aging and disease are not synonymous. In fact, the aging body can accomplish most, if not all, of the functions of its youth; the difference being that it may take longer, require more motivation, and be less precise.

Teaching Strategies

— Glossary terms

activities of daily living

cerumen

dementia

functional assessment

gerantology

longitudinal studies

micturition

presbycusis

programmed change theory

stochastic theories of aging

xerosis

— Other teaching strategies

Have students conduct a functional assessment on an older adult and do a drug history.

Examination questions

1. Percentiles, which are often used to evaulate a child's assessment data, represent the:

   a. the number of standard deviations above and below the mean
   - b. the percentage of values for the population that are above and below a certain number

2. The embryonic period:

   a. begins at the time of conception and continues through the second week of gestation
   - b. begins with the second week of gestation and continues through the 8th week
   c. begins with the second week of gestation and continues through the twelfth week
   d. begins with the ninth week of gestation and continues until birth

3. An infant is considered premature if it is born before the end of the:

   a. 28th week
   b. 30th week
   - c. 37th week
   d. 40th week

4. Small for gestational age denotes an infant with a birth weight that is less than

   a. 1 standard deviation or the 20th percentile
   - b. 2 standard deviations or the 10th percentile
   c. 3 standard deviations or the 30th percentile

5. Proportional or symetrical intrauterine growth retardation is usually related to events that occur:

   - a. early in pregnancy
   b. later in pregnancy

6. Which one of the following occurs almost exclusively in premature infants as compared to full time infants

   - a. intraventricular hemorrhage
   b. sudden death syndrome
   c. brachial nerve plexus
   d. cephalohematoma

7. The most common cause of death in infants between 6 and 12 months is:

   a. birth defects
   b. infections
   c. sudden infant death syndrome
   - d. injuries

8. The toddler period extends from:

   a. 12 to 18 months
   - b. 18 to 36 months
   c. 26 to 60 months

9. Bowel and bladder sphincter control follows myelinization of the:

   a. cortex
   b. brain stem
   - c. spinal cord occurs

10. The leading cause of illness during late childhood is:

    a. measles
    b. otitis media
  ● c. respiratory tract infections
    d. gastrointestinal disorders

11. Which one of the following statements is true as it relates to physical changes that occur with aging:

    a. physical dysfunction due to disease is an expected part of the aging process
    b. physical disability is synonymous with aging
  ● c. the aging body can accomplish most of its youthful functions but it may take longer

12. The stochastic theories of aging maintain that aging results from:

    a. genetically programmed events
  ● b. an accumulation of random events

13. The decline in height that occurs with aging is most directly related to:

  ● a. compression of the vertebral column
    b. a decrease in limb length
    c. increased adipose tissue
    d. lack of exercise

14. Normal aging produces which of the following changes in heart function:

    a. a decrease in resting cardiac output
    b. a decrease in resting heart rate
  ● c. a decrease in maximal exercise heart rate
    d. a decrease in exercise stroke volume

15. Normal neurologic changes that occur with aging include:

    a. decreased cognitive abilities
    b. impaired language skills
    c. personality changes
  ● d. slowed reaction time and diminished relexes

16. The most common visual problem associated with aging is:

    a. hyperopia
    b. myopia
    c. cataracts
  ● d. presbyopia

17. Which one of the following respiratory functions decrease as a result of the normal aging process:

  ● a. vital capacity
    b. total lung volume
    c. residual volume

18. Functional assessment focuses on:

    a. disease conditions
  ● b. functional abilities
    c. age-related changes in physiologic function
    d. psychosocial functioning

19. Transient causes of incontinence include:

    a. stress incontinence
  ● b. medications
    c. urge incontinence
    d. detrusor muscle inactivity

20. Which one of the following tend to make diagnosis of depression more difficult in older persons:

  ● a. presence of accompanying illness that confuse the diagnosis
    b. absence of suicidal thinking
    c. lack of feelings of self, feelings of worthlessness, self reproach, or guilt that accompany depression
    d. failure to display typical depressive symptomatology

Alterations in Integrated Body Functions

Unit 3 provides examples of responses that rely on integration of multiple body systems. Health includes the ability to adapt to stress and to work, exercise, participate in leisure activities, and perform activities of daily living. To be able to adapt to stress and perform these activities requires that integrated body responses provide the body with sufficient physiologic and psychologic reserve and stamina.

Chapter 8

Stress and Adaptation

Chapter 8 focuses on stress and adaptation. It includes Hans Selye's definition of stress and the neural, endocrine, musculoskeletal, and immune system responses to stress. There is a discussion of the constancy of the internal environment and the general features of homeostasis as described in Walter Cannon's book, *Wisdom of the Human Body*. The discussion in the chapter emphasizes that adaptation and homeostasis are idealized concepts, and that internal environment does not always return to normal. Adaptation is affected by previous experience and learning, physiologic reserve, rapidity of onset, genetic endowment, age, health status, nutrition, and psychosocial factors. The chapter ends with a brief discussion of biofeedback, relaxation, and imagery.

Teaching strategies

—Overhead transparencies

Figure 8-1 can be used to illustrate pathways whereby stress exerts its effects.

—Glossary terms

adaptation

biofeedback

circadian

diurnal

electromyographic

electrodermal

entrainment

homeostasis

imagery

milieu interne

negative feedback

physiologic and anatomic reserve

social support

stress and stressor

zeitgebers

Chapter 9

Alterations in Activity Tolerance

Chapter 9 focuses on activity tolerance. The chapter is organized into three parts: (1) activity tolerance and work performance, (2) activity intolerance and fatigue, and (3) bedrest and immobility.

Teaching strategies

—Glossary terms

aerobic activity

deconditioning

ergometry

fast and slow twitch
  muscle fibers

fatigue

hydrostatic forces

metabolic
  equivalents (METS)

supine

Examination questions

1. According to Hans Selye, stress is:

   a. anxiety and psychological response to excessive demands
   b. the autonomic nervous responses to an event that is perceived as threatening
   - c. the nonspecific response of the body to any demand made on it
   d. anything that alters psychological homeostasis

2. Specific stress responses are designed to:

   a. alert an individual to the presence of a stressor
   - b. maintain or reestablish homeostasis
   c. reduce anxiety
   d. overcome the stressor

3. In the central nervous system integration of the stress response, the thalamus:

   a. modulates mental alertness, autonomic system activity, and skeletal muscle tone
   - b. functions in sorting out and distributing sensory input
   c. modulates the function of the endocrine and autonomic nervous system
   d. is involved in the emotional components of the response

4. Which one of the following statements is true as it relates to the process of adaptation and its influence on body function during periods of stress:

   a. adaptation is most efficient when stress is suddenly induced
   - b. adaptation involves the whole person
   c. adaptation is most effective when the number of mechanisms available for the adaptive process are limited
   d. adaptation is always the same regardless of the type of stress that is encountered

5. The increased muscle tension that occurs with stress is a manifestation of increased activity of the:

   a. autonomic nervous system
   - b. reticular activation system
   c. hypothalamic-pituitary system
   d. motor cortex

6. Alterations in immune function that occur as the result of the stress response are thought to be at least partially related to:

   a. increased exposure to microorganisms due to ineffective coping behaviors
   b. increased anxiety and autonomic nervous system function
   - c. increased levels of corticosteroid hormones
   d. depression and lack of sleep

7. Which one of the following statements is characteristic of Walter B. Cannon's propositions about the general features of homeostasis:

    a. homeostasis depends on a single regulating system
    b. the constancy of the internal environment that represents homeostasis is regulated by a series of closed systems
    • c. any tendency toward change in the constancy of the internal environment is automatically met with factors that resist change
    d. homeostasis functions independent of organized self-government

8. The essential components of a homeostatic control system include:

    • a. a sensor, a comparator, and an effector
    b. a sensor, an amplifying system, and an effector
    c. a sensor and an effector
    d. a sensor, a comparator, and an error detection system

9. Synchronization of the biological clock with environmental influences is called:

    a. zietgebers
    • b. entrainment
    c. circadian rhythms
    d. free-running conditions

10. In persons with a normal sleep-wake cycle, serum cortisol levels are highest at:

    • a. 8 am to 9 am
    b. 12 noon
    c. 8 pm to 9 pm
    d. midnight

11. Exercise differs from actitivity in that:

    • a. exercise produces overall conditioning of the body
    b. exercise requires movement
    c. exercise requires energy expenditure

12. Muscle strength refers to:

    a. range of movement of joints
    • b. ability of muscle groups to produce force against resistance

13. Slow twitch muscle fibers play a major role in:

    • a. prolonged exercise or endurance activity
    b. activity that require short bursts of intense activity

14. Which statement is true regarding the cardiovascular responses to exercise:

    • a. heart rate rises immediately and continues to rise until a plateau is reached
    b. cardiac output rises solely due to an increase in heart rate
    c. systolic and diastolic undergo equal increases
    d. blood is diverted from the gas exchange portion of the pulmonary circulation to the skeletal muscles in the system circulation

15. Metabolic equivalents (METS) are commonly used to express workload for various stages of work. One MET is equivalent to the energy expended:

    a. during walking
    b. during eating
    c. during sleeping
    • d. in a resting position

16. The Borg exertion scale, measures exertion through the use of a person's:

    • a. report of perceived exertion
    b. heart rate response
    c. length of time and level of exercise
    d. blood pressure response

17. Which one of the following is characteristic of fatigue:

• a. fatigue is a subjective experience
   b. fatigue is always a physical experience
   c. fatigue is always relieved by rest or sleep

18. Chronic fatigue syndrome is characterized by fatigue that has been present for:

   a. 1 month
   b. 3 months
• c. 6 months
   d. 12 months

19. The direct antigravity effects of bedrest include:

• a. pooling of blood in the lower extremities
   b. decreased metabolic activity 12 noon
   c. decreased venous return to the heart
   d. decreased heart rate

20. The glucose intolerance that occurs with bedrest is thought to result from:

   a. increased glucose intake
   b. decreased filtering of glucose in the kidneys
   c. increased glucose concentration due to decreased extracellular fluid
• d. induced insulin resistance

Alterations in Body Defenses

Unit 4 focuses on body defenses that assist the body in dealing with stress, maintaining health, and preventing disease. Thermal regulating mechanisms (Chapter 10) protect against excess body heat production and extreme changes in environmental temperature. The skin (Chapter 11) serves as an interface between the internal and external environment; it prevents the loss of body fluids and protects against the entry of harmful environmental agents. Inflammation and immune system (Chapters 13) aids in tissue repair and defends against infectious organisms (Chapter 12). In concert with the inflammatory response, the immune system localizes the effects of injury and facilitates healing. The clotting system (Chapter 17) controls bleeding, localizes inflammatory lesions, and prevents the spread of infection. The content in Unit 4 focuses on both normal function of the body defense systems and disease processes that occur as a result of altered function. Chapter 12 focuses on altered immune responses, 13 is devoted to acquired immunodeficiency syndrome (AIDS), and Chapter 16 includes content on disorders of white blood cells and lymphoid tissue.

Chapter 10

Alterations in Temperature Regulation

Chapter 10 focuses on body temperature regulation and alterations in body temperature. Body temperature reflects the difference between heat gain which results from metabolic processes and occurs largely in the core tissues of the body, and heat loss which occurs largely at the interface between the skin and the external environment. Body temperature is regulated by the thermoregulatory center in the hypothalamus. The chapter emphasizes the difference between fever and hyperthermia; with fever caused by a change in the set-point of the thermoregulatory center and hyperthermia caused by extreme exercise, increased environmental temperature, and inadequate transport and dissipation of core heat due to fluid and electrolyte disorders. Because fever is often the first sign of serious drug reactions, descriptions of drug fever and neuroleptic malignant syndromes are provided in this chapter. The heart rate also provides essential information about the cause of fever; therefore, the relationship between heart rate and temperature elevation are discussed. For example, in the fever associated with Legionnaire's disease and drug fever the heart rate is often slower than anticipated, while in pulmonary embolism it is often higher than anticipated. Hypothermia is described as a core temperature less than 35°C and can be categorized as mild, moderate, and severe. The manifestations and treatment of hypothermia are discussed.

Teaching strategies

—Glossary terms

anorexia	hypothermia
antipyretic	hyperthermia
arthralgia	intermittent fever
conduction	neuroleptic
convection	pilomotor muscle
core temperature	prodrome
defervescence	pyrexia
delirium	pyrogen
evaporation	radiation
fatigue	recurrent fever
flush	relapsing fever
heat syncope	remittent fever

—Other teaching strategies

A. Develop a display of different types of thermometers, including one that could be used to measure the temperature of a person with hypothermia. Have students discuss the advantages and disadvantages of different thermometers and temperature taking sites (e.g., mouth, rectum, esophagus, and tympanic membrane) for measuring body temperature.

B. Discuss methods of reducing body temperature in hyperthermic conditions associated with exercise. Most classes will have runners or others who engage in sports that have the potential for inducing hyperthermia. Have the students discuss the difference between heat cramps, heat exhaustion, and heat stroke. Refer students to the references on face fanning as a method of emergency treatment for heat exhaustion "in the field," and have them explain the physiology involved (p. 102).

C. Have students discuss the principles underlying the use of tepid sponge baths and a cooling mattress to reduce body temperature in individuals with fever and hyperthermia. Discuss how chills and shivering induced by the cooling procedures influence treatment effectiveness.

Chapter 11

Alterations in Skin Function and Integrity

Chapter 11 focuses on structure of the skin and alterations in skin function and integrity that occur throughout the lifespan. There is a description of developmental skin problems, rashes associated with childhood, adolescent skin disorders, skin problems of the elderly, and skin problems specific to blacks. The chapter contains information about photosensitivity and sunburn, as well as insect bites, vectors, ticks, and parasites. Pressure ulcers, which involve both skin and the underlying tissue and result from impairment of local blood flow are presented in Chapter 18.

Teaching strategies

—Overhead transparencies

Chapter 8 is heavily illustrated with figures that depict various skin diseases and although these are difficult to reproduce as overheads, students can refer to them in their book.

Instructors may be able to obtain colored slides of skin lesions from local sources.

Figure 11-1 provides a three-dimensional view of skin structures.

—Glossary terms

apocrine glands	excoriation
blister	eczema
bulla	fissure
callus	hemangioma
crust	impetigo
dermis	keloid
eccrine gland	keratinized cells
epidermis	keratoses
erosion	lentigines
eruption	lesion

lichenification	pediculosis
macule	photosensitivity
melanin	plaque
melanoma	pustule
Mongolian spots	ulcer
nevus	vesicle
nodule	vitiligo
papule	wheal
patch	

—Other teaching strategies

A. Have students examine over-the-counter dermatologic preparations that are used in treatment of skin disorders such as acne, and explain their actions.

Chapter 12

Mechanisms of Infectious Disease

Chapter 12 is intended for students who have not had a microbiology course, or who need to review the content. The chapter includes a discussion of terminology used in microbiology, agents that cause infectious disease, the epidemiology of infectious disease, portals of entry, and symptomatology. Included in the chapter is a discussion of adherence factors which are becoming increasingly important in explaining the occurrence of infection. This content describes factors that predispose individuals to urinary tract infections, which is covered in Chapter 31. The chapter also includes a discussion of methods used in the diagnosis and treatment of infectious disease. The content in this chapter will help students understand the content in Chapter 10 (Inflammation and Repair), Chapter 13 (Acquired Immunodeficiency Syndrome), and Chapter 38 (Sexually Transmitted Diseases).

Teaching strategies

—Overhead transparency

Figure 12-1 Shows the structure of viruses.

Figure 12-2 Illustrates the many consequences of viral infection in host cells.

Figure 12-5 shows the stages of primary infections as they relate to severity of symptoms and numbers of infectious agents.

—Glossary terms

anaerobes	flagella
colonization	incidence
commensalism	incubation period
culture	microflora
epidemiology	mutualism
eukaryotic cells	opportunistic infection
fimbriae	

parasites   prevalence   saprophyte   symptomatology
pili   prokaryotes   serology   virulence

Chapter 13

Inflammation and Immunity

Chapter 13 discusses inflammation and immunity. The first part of the chapter presents inflammation as a normal response that prepares injured tissue for wound healing and reparative processes. Similar to the stress response covered in Chapter 8, inflammation involves a sequence of specific physiologic behaviors that occur in response to a nonspecific agent. The chapter includes a discussion of acute and chronic inflammation and a description of mediators and inflammatory exudates.

The second part of the chapter provides an overview of the immune system. This chapter forms the basis for understanding content in Chapters 14 and 15, and for immune mechanisms presented in other chapters of the book. The presentation of content in this chapter has been simplified to facilitate understanding by students who do not have an extensive background in genetics and biochemistry. There is a discussion of the organs and cells of the immune system, differentiation of T and B-lymphocytes, macrophage function, antigen specific functions of the T and B-lymphocytes, antigen nonspecific immune mechanisms, and the major histocompatibility complex antigens and the ability of the immune system to recognize self from nonself.

Teaching strategies

—Overhead transparencies

Figure 13-1 can be used to illustrate the white blood cells that are involved in the inflammatory response.

Figure 13-6 more fully describes the macrophage in presentation of the antigen to the immune cells and in facilitating the interaction between B-cells and T-cells.

—Glossary Terms

abscess

antibody

antigen

cellulitis

chemotaxis

complement

cytokines

cytotoxic

diapedesis

engulfment

endogenous

eosinophil

epitope

exogenous

exudate (membranous, purulent, serous, suppurative)

hapten

human leukocyte antigens (HLA)

immunity

immunoglobulin

interferons

leukocyte (band, basophil, monocyte, neutrophil, polymorphonuclear, stab)

leukotrienes

lymphocyte

lymphokines

macrophage

major histocompatibility complex (MHC)

microphages

phagocytosis

plasma proteases

proliferation

prostaglandins

pyogenic

opsonization

regeneration

reticuloendothelial system

serosanguinous

Chapter 14

Alterations in the Immune Response

Chapter 14 describes alterations in immune function. The discussion in the chapter focuses on primary and secondary immunodeficiency states, including disorders of complement and phagocyte function, allergy and hypersensitivity, and autoimmune disease, using systemic lupus erythematosus as a model. Acquired immunodeficiency due to HIV infection is discussed in Chapter 13. Type I IgE-mediated, type II IgG- and IgM-mediated cytotoxic, type III IgG- and IgM-mediated antigen antibody complex, and type IV cell-mediated responses are discussed in this chapter. Because of the increased use of organ transplantation a discussion of transplant rejection was included in this chapter.

Teaching strategies

—Overhead transparencies

Figure 14-1 shows stem cells to mature immunoglobulin-secreting plasma cells.

Figures 14-4, 14-5, 14-6, and 14-7 can be used to illustrate allergic and hypersensitivity responses.

—Glossary terms

allergy

angioneurotic edema

antitoxin

atopic

autoimmune

desensitization

eczematous

graft-versus-host disease

host-versus-graft disease

hypersensitivity reaction

hypogammaglobuline mia

idiopathic

immune complex

intradermal

LE cells

mast cells

rhinitis

self-tolerance

superantigen

Chapter 15

Acquired Immunodeficiency Syndrome (AIDS)

Because of the rapid increase in the incidence and prevalence of human immunodeficiency virus (HIV) infection and acquired immunodeficiency disease (AIDS), an entire chapter has been devoted to this disease. The chapter begins with a history of the AIDS epidemic, and includes a discussion of the transmission of the HIV infection, as well as the general principles of universal precautions. The pathophysiology of AIDS, prevention, its clinical manifestations, diagnostic procedures, and management are discussed. The chapter includes a discussion of the vertical transmission of HIV infection from mother to infant and AIDS in children.

Teaching strategies

—Glossary terms

candidiasis

enzyme-linked immunoassay (EIA OR ELISA)

human immunodeficiency virus (HIV)

Kaposi's sarcoma

lymphadenopathy

Pneumocystis carinii

retrovirus

universal precautions

wasting disease

—Other teaching strategies

A. Discuss the current blood tests for AIDS and discuss their effectiveness. If appropriate, have students obtain information from their local blood center related to measures used to prevent AIDS transmission through blood products. Among methods that students may want to discuss are cell salvage methods that are used during surgery and autotransfusion methods.

B. Have students read and report on current newspaper and journal articles on the AIDS epidemic. Discuss the importance of the use of the universal precautions by health professionals. Have students obtain information on OSHA regulations for protection of health care workers and the impact on health care costs.

Chapter 16

Disorders of White Blood Cells and Lymphoid Tissues

Chapter 16 focuses on disorders of granulocytes and proliferative disorders of white blood cells and lymphoid tissues. The chapter provides a description of the multipotential hemopoietic stem cell, and traces granulocyte production. Chapter content includes a discussion of leukopenia and agranulocytosis, acute and chronic infectious mononucleosis, acute and chronic lymphocytic and monocytic leukemia, lymphomas and Hodgkin's disease, and multiple myeloma.

Teaching strategies
—Glossary terms

agranulocytopenia	heteroantibodies
agranulocytosis	lethargy
aplastic anemia	leukopenia
Bence Jones proteins	lymphoid tissue
blast cell	multiple myeloma
ecchymosis	myelocytic
epistaxis	petechiae
Epstein-Barr virus	Reed-Sternberg cell
gingival	splenomegaly
hepatomegaly	

Chapter 17

Alterations in Blood Coagulation and Hemostasis

Chapter 17 focuses on hemostasis; it incorporates a discussion of platelets and coagulation factors including von Willebrand's factor. The chapter is organized into hypercoagulability states and bleeding diatheses including thrombocytopenia, hemophilia, and von Willebrand's disease. A brief discussion of disseminated intravascular clotting (DIC) is included in this chapter. The use of cryoprecipitate in treatment of hemophilia is discussed. There is also a brief discussion of the thrombolytic agents used in treatment of myocardial infarction (Chapter 21).

Teaching strategies

—Overhead transparencies

Figure 17-1 illustrates the step in the coagulation process.

Figure 17-12 can be used to illustrate the intrinsic and extrinsic coagulation pathways. This diagram is useful in describing the sites where heparin and coumadin exert their effects.

—Glossary terms

cryoprecipitate

disseminated intravascular clotting (DIC)

abruptio placenta

fibrin

fibrinogen

fibrinolysis

thrombolytic agents

petechiae

purpura

thrombocytopenia

thrombopoietin

von Willebrand's factor

Examination questions

1. Mechanisms of body heat production include:

   • a. shivering and increased cellular metabolism
   b. shivering, contraction of the pilomotor muscles, and assumption of the huddle position
   c. vasoconstriction of the skin vessels and contraction of the pilomotor muscles
   d. vasodilation of the skin vessels and activation of the sympathetic nervous system

2. Radiation involves:

   a. heat transfer through the circulation of air currents
   • b. heat transfer through the air or a vacuum
   c. the transfer of heat from one molecule to another
   d. the use of heat to vaporize water

3. A remittent fever is one in which the temperature:

   • a. returns to normal at least once in every 24 hours
   b. does not return to normal but varies a few degrees in either direction
   c. remains above normal with minimal variations
   d. returns to normal for one or more days between episodes of fever

4. Fever differs from hyperthermia in terms of:

   a. the presence of an increase in body temperature above the normal range
   • b. the upward displacement of hypothalamic set point for temperature control
   c. the presence of an elevated heart rate
   d. an increase in body metabolism

5. Which one of the following should be avoided when cooling is used as a treatment for reducing body temperature in a person with fever:

   a. rapid reduction in body temperature
   b. sweating
   • c. shivering
   d. vasodilation

6. Heat cramps result from:

   a. shivering that occurs
   b. increased metabolism of the affected muscle groups
   • c. sodium losses due to sweating and drinking tap water
   d. the effect of heat on muscle proteins

7. Drug fever should be suspected whenever there is:

   a. a low-grade temperature elevation in someone who is taking medications
 • b. an elevated temperature that is unexpected and occurs despite improvement in the condition for which the drug was prescribed
   c. a late afternoon elevation in temperature in someone who is taking medications
   d. the condition causing a fever persists despite drug therapy

8. Neuroleptic malignant hyperthermia is usually accompanied by:

   a. bradycardia and hypertension
 • b. muscle rigidity and autonomic nervous system dysfunction
   c. muscle paralysis and diarrhea
   d. apprehension and decreased respiratory rate

9. Oral temperatures are usually not recommended during hypothermia because:

   a. oral thermometers that register below 95° are not available on the market
   b. respiratory rate is decreased in hypothermia and this will alter the oral temperature
 • c. vasoconstriction and sluggish blood flow impair the movement of core heat to the oral mucosa
   d. positioning of the thermometer is difficult because of the intense shivering that is present

10. The objective of active core rewarming in a person with severe hypothermia is to:

    a. produce gradual rewarming of all of the structures of the body
    b. reduce discomfort by rapidly rewarming the core structures
 • c. minimize complications associated with returning cold extremity blood to an unwarmed heart by initial rewarming of the core structures
    d. return skin temperature to normal as rapidly as possible

11. A fever that is not accompanied by the normally expected increase in heart rate is associated with:

    a. hyperthyroidism
 • b. drug fever
    c. bacterial infections
    d. viral infections

12. The melanocytes are found in which of the skin structures:

 • a. epidermis
    b. dermis
    c. basement membrane zone
    d. sebaceous glands

13. The sweat glands and pilomotor muscles are innervated by:

    a. the parasympathetic nervous system
 • b. the sympathetic nervous system
    c. the motoneurons that innervate the skeletal muscles

14. The sweat glands and hair follicles receive their blood supply and innervation from the:

 • a. epidermis
    b. dermis
    c. subcutaneous tissues

15. Sweating that contributes to temperature regulation is a function of the:

 • a. eccrine sweat glands
    b. apocrine sweat glands

16. A papule is a small:

    a. flat circumscribed skin lesion
    • b. solid elevated skin lesion
    c. superficial skin elevation that is filled with fluid
    d. elevated pus-filled lesion

17. In an infant, prickly heat results from:

    a. inflammation of the hair follicles
    b. damage to the keratinocytes
    • c. obstruction and rupture of the sweat glands
    d. irritation of the pilomotor unit

18. Which one of the following skin disorders seen in elderly persons is considered a pre-malignant lesion:

    a. seborrheic keratosis
    • b. actinic keratosis
    c. senile lentigines
    d. telangiectases

19. Which one of the following is characterized by the presence of postauricular, subauricular, and cervical lymph node adenopathy:

    a. roseola infantum
    b. rubeola
    • c. rubella
    d. scarlet fever

20. Which one of the following is caused by a virus:

    • a. warts
    b. impetigo
    c. athlete's foot
    d. psoriasis

21. The disintegration of the nail in tinea unguium or onchomycosis is caused by:

    • a. a fungal enzyme that digests keratin
    b. a metabolic end-product of fungal growth that impairs mitosis in keratin cells
    c. homeostatic mechanisms that reduce blood flow to the infected nail
    d. liberation of lactic acid by the infecting fungus

22. Acne is a disorder of the:

    a. keratinocytes
    b. apocrine sweat glands
    • c. pilosebaceous unit
    d. melanocytes

23. Herpes zoster is characterized by:

    • a. lesions that are restricted to skin areas supplied by a single dorsal root ganglia
    b. recurrent lesions of skin and mucous membranes
    c. recurrent lesions of genital region
    d. generalized herpetic lesions

24. Malignant melanomas are usually characterized by:

    a. scaly, keratotic slightly elevated lesions with an irregular border
    b. elevated pigmented hairy lesions
    c. small, smooth shiny nodule that enlarges over time
    • d. slightly raised dark lesions, that frequently advance to include mottled shades of red, white, and blue

25. Colonization refers to:

    • a. the presence or multiplication of a living organism on or within a host
    b. the harmless inhabitation of bacteria on or within a host
    c. an interaction between a host and a microorganism that is mutually beneficial
    d. an interaction between a host and a microorganism which only benefits the microorganism

26. Unicellular organisms that lack an organized nucleus are referred to as:

● a. prokaryotes
   b. eukaryotes

27. Fungi that reproduce by the budding process are classified as:

● a. yeasts
   b. molds

28. Examples of ectoparasites include:

   a. tapeworms and fluxes
● b. lice and fleas
   c. yeasts and molds
   d. rickettsias and chlamydia

29. Incidence refers to the number of:

● a. new cases of a disease
   b. number of active cases that are present at any given time

30. The prodromal stage of an infectious disease is characterized by:

● a. a pathogen which begins replication without symptom production
   b. appearance of symptoms
   c. maximum proliferation and dissemination of the pathogen
   d. containment and progressive elimination of the pathogen

31. Nosocomial infections are those that:

   a. are spread from the mother to the infant during gestation
● b. develop in hospitalized patients
   c. are passed from animals to humans
   d. are spread by biting arthropods

32. An example of a disease or disease state caused by exotoxins is:

● a. diphtheria
   b. endotoxic shock
   c. gonorrhea
   d. measles

33. Penicillins exert their therapeutic effect by:

   a. inhibiting bacterial protein synthesis
   b. interrupting of nucleic acid synthesis
● c. inhibiting bacterial cell wall synthesis
   d. interfering with normal pathogen metabolism

34. Inflammation can best be described as:

   a. the body's response to an infectious process
   b. an abnormal event that accompanies selected disease processes
● c. a normal body response to cell and tissue injury
   d. a disease process that is accompanied by fever

35. The transudation of fluid that occurs at the site of an acute inflammatory response is of benefit to the host because it:

● a. dilutes the noxious agent
   b. increases the absorption of the noxious agent
   c. allows lymphocytes to enter the area
   d. produces a local increase in temperature

36. The local heat that occurs during an inflammatory response is the result of:

   a. substances liberated from injured cells
● b. increased blood flow
   c. swelling
   d. leukocytosis

37. The white blood cell that has the greatest rate of increase during a bacterial infection is the:

   a. eosinophil
   b. lymphocyte
   c. basophil
● d. neutrophil

38. Chemotaxis involves the:

- a. attraction of leukocytes to an injurious agent
  b. ameboid-type movement that propel white blood cells through the capillary wall and tissues spaces
  c. engulfment and degradation of bacteria and cellular debris by the white blood cells
  d. the increase in white blood cell numbers that occurs during the inflammatory response

39. A thin and watery exudate that contains red blood cells is called a:

- a. serous exudate
  b. purulent exudate
  c. fibrinous exudate
  d. serosanguinous exudate

40. The function of the immune system is:

  a. limited to the destruction of infectious agents
- b. to destroy foreign agents and prevent the development and growth of abnormal cells
  c. to destroy agents and cells that are recognized as both self and non-self
  d. limited to the use of antibodies to neutralize and destroy antigens

41. Specific immune mechanisms include protection afforded by:

  a. the complement system
  b. phagocytosis
- c. cell-mediated immunity
  d. natural killer cells

42. Which one of the following is an example of active immunity:

  a. protection against infections that is passed from mother to infant through the placenta
- b. protection afforded by the flu vaccine
  c. protection afforded against hepatitis by an injection of pooled gamma globulin
  d. protection afforded to infant from a mother's breast milk

43. Differentiation of T lymphocytes occurs in the:

  a. bone marrow
  b. spleen
- c. thymus
  d. lymphatic system

44. Which type of lymphocyte plays the greatest role in the development of humoral immunity:

  a. T-lymphocytes
- b. B-lymphocytes

45. Which one of the following classes of immunoglobulins cross the placenta:

  a. IgA
  b. IgE
- c. IgG
  d. IgM

46. Class I major histocompatibility complex (MHC) antigens are found on:

  a. immune cells
- b. all nucleated cells of the body
  c. bone marrow cells
  d. kidney cells

47. The macrophages:

    a. act as killer cells to destroy cancer cells

 • b. capture and process antigen and present it to the lymphocytes

    c. are responsible for removal of injurious agents during an acute inflammatory response

    d. produce a chemical substance that attracts white blood cells to an area of acute inflammation

48. Which one of the following types of immunoglobulins is involved in allergic and hypersensitivity responses:

    a. IgA

 • b. IgE

    c. IgG

    d. IgM

49. The protection against polio that is afforded by the oral sabin is in the form of:

 • a. IgA antibodies

    b. IgE antibodies

    c. IgG antibodies

    d. IgM antibodies

50. The lymph nodes:

 • a. assist in removing foreign materials from the lymph channels and are centers for immune cell proliferation

    b. contain the precursor cells of the immune system

    c. are the site where lymphocytes differentiate into either T cells or B cells

    d. serve to disseminate antigens and injurious agents

51. The complement system could best be described as a system of:

    a. blood cells that are needed for the immune response

 • b. inactive circulating precursor proteins that function as a mediator of humoral immunity

    c. blood proteins that function as chemotactic agents

    d. phagocytic cells that are activated by humoral immune mechanisms

52. A secondary cause of impaired cellular immunity is:

    a. loss of immunoglobulins due to the nephrotic syndrome

 • b. Hodgkin's disease

    c. multiple myeloma

    d. decreased immunoglobulin synthesis due to lymphoma

53. The age at which infants are usually able to produce adequate amounts of gamma globulin is:

    a. at birth

    b. 2 to 3 months of age

 • c. 5 to 6 months of age

    d. 12 to 16 months of age

54. Type I (atopic) hypersensitivity immune responses include:

 • a. hay fever and bronchial asthma

    b. transplant rejection

    c. transfusion reactions

    d. serum sickness

55. The mediators involved in allergic responses are released from:

 • a. mast cells or basophils

    b. plasma cells

    c. macrophages

    d. the antigen

56. The immunoglobulins that are responsible for activation of complement in type II immune responses are:

    a. IgA and IgE
    b. IgE and IgG
  • c. IgG and IgM
    d. IgD and IgM

57. The symptoms of serum sickness include:

    a. running nose and bronchospasm
  • b. skin rash and fever
    c. generalized edema and difficulty breathing
    d. anaphylaxis and shock

58. The time period between exposure to an offending antigen and the manifestations of serum sickness is usually:

    a. 2 to 3 hours
    b. 2 to 3 days
  • c. 7 to 10 days
    d. 2 to 3 months

59. One of the most common causes of serum sickness is:

    a. pollens
    b. food allergies
  • c. drugs
    d. molds

60. A chronic transplant rejection response is caused by:

    a. the presence of existing recipient antibodies to the graft
    b. a humoral immune response
  • c. a cell-mediated immune response

61. Graft-versus host disease occurs most commonly in which type of transplant:

    a. kidney
    b. liver
    c. heart
  • d. bone marrow

62. AIDS is caused by the:

  • a. human immunodeficiency virus
    b. herpes virus
    c. papilloma virus
    d. adenovirus

63. Replication of a retrovirus involves:

  • a. translation of the viral RNA into DNA prior to insertion into the host chromosome
    b. insertion of the viral DNA directly into the host chromosome
    c. insertion of the viral RNA directly into the host chromosome
    d. translation of viral DNA into RNA prior to insertion into the host chromosome

64. AIDS is spread through:

    a. blood, sexual contact, sweat, and gastrointestinal secretions
  • b. blood, sexual contact, maternal-placental circulation, and breast milk
    c. blood, sexual contact, fomites, and sweat
    d. sputum, sexual contact, gastro-intestinal secretions, and blood

65. The AIDS virus directly infects the:

    a. neutrophils
  • b. CD4 lymphocytes
    c. CD8 lymphocytes
    d. B lymphocytes

66. Opportunistic infections are:

  • a. infections involving usually harmless microorganisms that develop in persons' compromised immune function
    b. hospital acquired infections
    c. infections that develop in persons who have not been immunized against or previously exposed to a particular microorganism
    d. hypersensitivity reactions that develop in persons who are predisposed to allergies

67. Universal precautions are designed to prevent exposure to infectious agents that are present in:

    a. the air
    • b. blood, semen, and vaginal secretions
    c. sweat, tears, and nasal secretions
    d. gastrointestinal tract secretions

68. The diagnostic blood tests for HIV infection detect:

    a. the virus
    • b. antibody to the AIDS virus
    c. white blood cells that are infected with the virus
    d. levels of reverse transcriptase which is required for viral replication

69. A positive antibody test in an infant indicates:

    a. that the infant is infected with the HIV virus
    • b. a perinatally exposed infant with maternal antibodies

70. The "window phase" of HIV infection refers to the period of time:

    a. between infection and the acute mononucleosis-like symptoms
    b. between infection and appearance of initial symptoms
    • c. between infection and detectable antibody levels
    d. between exacerbations and remissions of the disease

71. The most common cause of agranulocytosis is:

    a. a congenital defect in granulocyte production
    • b. drug-related suppression of bone marrow function or increased granulocyte destruction
    c. neoplasms involving the bone marrow
    d. inflammatory process that cause increased removed of granulocytes

72. In the course of acute infectious mononucleosis, the Epstein-Barr virus invades:

    • a. B-lymphocytes
    b. T-lymphocytes
    c. macrophages
    d. bone marrow stem cells

73. Which one of the following types of leukemia has its peak incidence in early childhood:

    • a. acute lymphocytic leukemia
    b. chronic lymphocytic leukemia
    c. acute myelocytic leukemia
    d. chronic myelocytic leukemia

74. The warning signs of acute leukemia are:

    a. bone pain, weight loss, fever, and headache
    • b. fatigue, paleness, weight loss, repeated infections, easy bruising and other bleeding disorders
    c. swollen lymph nodes, weight gain, headache, and easy bruising
    d. bleeding, abdominal pain, headache, and fever

75. Increased vulnerability to infection that occurs in persons with leukemia is caused by:

    a. subperiosteal bone infiltration and bone-marrow expansion
    b. anemia
    • c. immaturity of white blood cells
    d. generalized lymphadenopathy

76. Hodgkin's disease is a malignant neoplasm of:

    a. bone marrow
    b. spleen
    • c. lymphatic structures
    d. blood cells

77. Signs of disease spread in persons with Hodgkin's disease include:

    a. bleeding, abdominal pain, and headache
    ● b. fatigue, fever, night sweats, and unexplained weight loss
    c. headache and neurological manifestations
    d. elevated blood pressure and bone pain

78. Multiple myeloma is a malignancy of the:

    a. T-lymphocytes
    b. B-lymphocytes
    c. lymphatic system
    ● d. plasma cells

79. An early manifestation of multiple myeloma is:

    ● a. bone pain
    b. headache
    c. neurological manifestations
    d. kidney failure

80. The first step of hemostasis is:

    a. development of an insoluble fibrin clot
    b. formation of a platelet plug
    c. clot retraction
    ● d. vessel spasm

81. Von Willebrand's factor is directly involved in:

    ● a. platelet adhesion
    b. platelet aggregation
    c. formation of the fibrin clot
    d. clot dissolution

82. The fibrinolytic agents that are used in treatment of a heart attack act by:

    a. preventing blood clot formation
    ● b. activating the physiologic proenzyme for the clot dissolution process
    c. digesting the blood clot
    d. preventing platelet aggregation

83. Thrombocytopenia results from the deficiency of which one of the following:

    a. prothrombin
    b. fibrinogen
    c. thrombin
    ● d. platelets

84. The main action of aspirin in terms of bleeding disorders is related to:

    a. platelet production
    b. platelet adhesion
    ● c. platelet aggregation

85. Stasis of blood flow increases the risk of blood clotting via the coagulation system because of:

    ● a. reduced clearance of activated clotting factors
    b. increased levels of deoxygenated hemoglobin
    c. increased turbulence of flow
    d. decreased pressure

86. Hemophilia A results from a deficiency of:

    a. thrombocytes
    b. von Willebrand's factor
    ● c. factor VIII
    d. factor IX

87. Disseminated intravascular clotting (DIC) is characterized by:

    ● a. formation of microemboli, consumption of clotting factors, loss of platelets, clot dissolution, and bleeding
    b. formation of microemboli and consumption of clotting factors
    c. consumption of clotting factors and bleeding
    d. formation of microemboli

88. The anticoagulant drug Coumarin (coumadin) acts by:

   a. inhibiting the thrombin-mediated conversion of fibronogen to fibrin
   b. impairing platelet adhesion
   c. inhibiting the production of von Willebrand's factor
   • d. impairing the synthesis of vitamin K dependent clotting factors

89. The anticoagulant drug heparin acts by:

   • a. inhibiting the action of thrombin on fibrinogen
   b. interrupting the intrinsic coagulation pathway
   c. inactivating the calcium-dependent steps in the coagulation pathway
   d. interfering with the synthesis of prothrombin

Alterations in Oxygenation of Tissues

Oxygenation of tissues requires a vehicle for oxygen transport (hemoglobin), a system that circulates oxygen and the end products of metabolism, and a system for gas exchange between the internal and external environments. Unit 5 is divided into 11 chapters. The first chapter describes both normal and altered red blood cell structure and function; Chapters 17 through 23 are concerned with the circulatory system; and Chapters 24 through 26 cover the respiratory system. When teaching the circulatory system it is always difficult to decide whether to begin with the heart or the blood vessels. In this case, the decision to begin with a discussion of blood vessels and blood flow was based on later application to the coronary circulation and on the effects that flow and pressure exert on the work demands of the heart. Because of its importance as a major health problem, a separate chapter (Chapter 19) was devoted to alterations in blood pressure (hypertension).

Chapter 18

The Red Blood Cell and Alterations in Oxygen Transport

The major function of the red blood cell, facilitated by the hemoglobin molecule, is the transport of oxygen. The hemoglobin molecule is composed of two pairs of structurally different polypeptide chains (an a chain and a b chain) attached to a heme unit which, in turn, surrounds an atom of iron that binds oxygen. Chapter 16 focuses on red blood cell structure, the life cycle of a red cell from its development in the bone marrow to its destruction in the spleen, liver, lymph nodes, or bone marrow. Among the red blood cell disorders discussed in the chapter are blood loss anemia, hemolytic anemias, nutritional anemias, anemia resulting from bone marrow depression, and polycythemia. A discussion of alterations in red cell function that occur in sickle cell anemia, the thalassemias, G6PD deficiency, and hemolytic disease of the newborn is included in the chapter. One of the unique features of this chapter is a discussion of transfusion therapy. There is a discussion of the advantages of component therapy in which a number of blood constituents are obtained from a single unit of blood.

Teaching strategies

—Overhead transparency

Figure 18-3 can be used to illustrate the life span of a red blood cell from its differentiation in the bone marrow to its release into the blood.

Chapter 19

The Circulatory System and Control of Blood Flow

Chapter 19 is designed to aid students in understanding content regarding blood flow and blood pressure in subsequent chapters in this unit; it describes the organization and function of the blood vessels as a system of distributing tubes (arteries), collecting tubes (veins), and an extensive system of thin vessels that facilitate the rapid exchange between the tissues and the vascular channels. A discussion of blood pressure control is included in Chapter 19 and a discussion of heart function is presented in Chapter 20. The chapter includes a discussion of the physics of blood flow and neural control and autoregulation of blood flow.

Teaching strategies

—Overhead transparencies

Figure 19-7 illustrates the similarities and differences between the structure of arteries and veins.

Figure 19-9 shows the capillary bed. Pictured in this figure are the arterioles that control the total peripheral resistance. This figure can also be used when discussing the

manner in which arterioles regulate total peripheral resistance (Chapter 21) and when discussing the effects of shock on flow in the microcirculation (Chapter 25).

—Glossary terms

artery

arteriole

atrial filling pressure

central circulation

collateral circulation

cross-sectional area

endothelium

energy (total,
  kinetic, potential)

hyperemia

laminar flow

lumen

microcirculation

peripheral
  circulation

pressure gradient

pressure wave

peripheral vascular
  resistance

turbulent flow

viscosity

wall tension

—Other teaching strategies

A. Have students demonstrate reactive hyperemia by putting pressure over a bony prominence such as the elbow or placing a hand in cold water.

Chapter 20

Alterations in Blood Flow

Chapter 20 focuses on alterations in blood flow. An introduction to conditions that impair blood flow precedes the discussion of specific disorders. Alterations in arterial flow include atherosclerosis, arterial aneurysms, acute arterial occlusion, Raynaud's phenomenon, and thromboangiitis obliterans. There is a discussion of blood lipids and assessment of arterial flow. Alterations in venous function is characterized by varicose veins, venous insufficiency, and venous thrombosis. The chapter ends with a discussion of impairment of local blood flow and pressure sores.

One of the key concepts that instructors will want to emphasize is that in order for blood to flow: arterial pressure must be greater than venous pressure and both arterial and venous pressure must be greater than surrounding tissue pressure. In the brain the surrounding pressure includes both the cerebrospinal fluid pressure and tissue pressure and in the lungs it includes the alveolar pressure. In compartment syndrome, elevating the arm may lower arterial pressure and thereby compromised muscle compartment perfusion. In the case of venous obstruction, elevating an extremity would tend to lower venous pressure and improve blood flow.

Teaching strategies

—Overhead transparencies

Figure 20-1 shows conditions that alter blood flow.

Figure 20-4 provides a schematic representation of the exogenous and endogenous lipoprotein and cholesterol transport.

Figure 20-5 can be used to illustrate the difference between a berry aneurysm, fusiform-type aneurysm, and a dissecting aneurysm.

—Glossary terms

aneurysm	hypercholesteremia
atheroma	Homan's sign
arteriosclerosis	thrombi
atherosclerosis	thrombolytic
chylomicrons	thromboangiitis obliterans
decubitus ulcer	
emboli	triglycerides
lipoproteins (high density and low density)	stasis dermatitis
	incompetent veins

Chapter 21

Alterations in Blood Pressure: Hypertension and Orthostatic Hypotension

Blood pressure represents the pressure force that is exerted in blood vessels. Although pressure contributes to the flow of blood throughout the circulatory system, it is customary to equate blood pressure with pressure in the systemic arteries. The mean arterial pressure represents the force needed to overcome the resistance in the systemic circulation and move the cardiac output from the left heart and return it to the right heart. Chapter 19 focuses on alterations in arterial blood pressure. The chapter is divided into three parts: control of blood pressure, hypertension, and orthostatic hypotension. In addition to essential and secondary forms of hypertension, this chapter provides a discussion of hypertension in pregnancy, in children, and in the elderly. There is a discussion of normal blood pressure changes that occur during infancy and childhood, pregnancy, and as a result of the aging process.

Teaching strategies

—Overhead transparencies

Figure 21-2 shows the cardiovascular events associated with systolic and diastolic blood pressure.

Figure 21-4 illustrates the control of blood pressure by the renin-angiotensin-aldosterone system.

—Glossary terms

adrenergic

angiotenisn-converting enzyme

atrial naturetic factor

auscultatory sounds

baroreceptors

catecholamines

cholinergic

coarctation

diastolic blood pressure

hydatidiform mole

hypertension

hypotension

Korotkoff sounds

orthostatic

pheochromocytoma

preeclampsia

pulse pressure

peripheral (systemic) vascular resistance

renin

renin-angiotensin mechanism

renovascular hypertension

systolic blood pressure

vasopressin

—Other teaching strategies

A. Have students: (1) measure the heart rate and blood pressure of a classmate in the supine position and after standing for two minutes; (2) use the blood pressure measurements to calculate the pulse pressure and mean arterial blood pressure.

B. Obtain a portable hand-grip for doing isometric exercise. Have students measure a classmate's blood pressure before performing isometric exercise and again after 1 and 2 minutes of squeezing the handgrip. Both systolic and diastolic blood pressure should rise. Other stresses can also be used to demonstrate the effect of activities of daily living on blood pressure.

Chapter 22

Control of Cardiac Function

Chapter 22 was designed to help the student understand normal heart function. The chapter includes a discussion of the embryonic development of the heart, the structure of the heart wall, heart valves and the directional control of blood flow, the conduction system and the electrical activity of the heart, the cardiac cycle, regulation of cardiac performance and factors affecting cardiac output, the coronary circulation, the metabolic demands of the heart, and the determinants of oxygen consumption. It is suggested that students read this chapter in preparation for understanding the content in Chapters 21 and 22.

Teaching strategies

—Overhead transparencies

Figure 22-1 illustrates the position of the heart and great vessels in the thorax. This figure emphasizes the fact that the heart and great vessels are in the thoracic cavity, and are exposed to the intrathoracic pressure changes that occur with respiratory maneuvers.

Figure 22-5 shows the valular structures of the heart and the directional flow of blood through the heart. This figure can also be used when discussing valvular defects.

Figure 22-7 depicts the conduction system of the heart along with the action potentials.

Figure 22-9 shows the relationship between the electrocardiogram and a ventricular action potential.

Figure 22-10 shows fast action potential response of the cardiac muscle cells and the slow response of the pacemaker and conduction tissues of the heart. It is suggested that this figure should be used in conjunction with Figure 22-7.

Figure 22-11 diagrams the action potential of a ventricular muscle cell showing the resting membrane potential, absolute refractory period, and relative refractory period. This figure will prove useful when discussing the origin and treatment of cardiac dysrhythmias.

Figure 22-12 depicts the events in the cardiac cycle including the relationship between the heart sounds, electrical events, ventricular volume, and pressure changes during systole and diastole.

Figure 22-13 shows the Starling ventricular function curve (top) along with the stretching of the actin and myosin filaments that accompany different left end diastolic volumes. This diagram should also prove useful when discussing heart failure.

—Glossary terms

afterload	intercalated disks
atria	myocardium
bundle of His	mitral valve
calcium channels	papillary muscles
cardiac cycle	pacemaker
cardiac output	preload
cardiac reserve	pericardium
chordae tendineae	Purkinje system
diastole	semilunar valves
ductus arteriosus	Starling's law of the heart
endocardium	
epicardium	stroke work
foramen ovale	stroke volume
inotropic	systole
isometric contraction	tricuspid valve
isovolumetric contraction	Valsalva's maneuver

Chapter 23

Alterations in Cardiac Function

Chapter 23, which focuses on common heart problems across the life-span, has been organized into seven sections: (1) disorders of the pericardium, (2) coronary heart disease, (3) disorders of cardiac rhythm and conduction, (4) diseases of the myocardium, (5) disorders of the endocardium, (6) valvular heart disease, and (7) congenital heart disease. Silent myocardial ischemia and recent developments in the use of thrombolytic therapy and percutaneous transluminal coronary artery angioplasty are included in the section on coronary heart disease. Because cardiac dysrhythmia and conduction defects are often described in terms of their electrocardiograph manifestations, a discussion of the electrocardiogram is used as an introduction to the section on disorders of cardiac rhythm and conduction.

Teaching strategies

—Overhead transparencies

Figure 23-2 shows the coronary arteries.

Figure 23-11 is a diagram of the electrocardiogram.

Figure 23-23 shows the fetal circulation and the fetal shunts (foramen ovale and ductus arteriosus)

Figure 23-24 depicts congenital heart defects and altered blood flow caused by these defects.

—Glossary terms

automaticity

aberrant

angina pectoris

bradycardia

bigeminy

cardiomyopathy

chorea

conductivity

cyanotic heart disease

dysrhythmias

echocardiography

ectopic pacemaker

electrocardiograph leads (bipolar and unipolar)

endocarditis

epistaxis

excitability

fibrillation

flutter

heart block (first, second, and third degree)

intramyocardial

Kussmaul's sign

metabolic equivalents (METs)

myocarditis

nuclear imaging

pericarditis

percutaneous transluminal coronary angioplasty

pericardial effusion

phonocardiography

preductal

polyarthritis

postductal

pulsus paradoxus

re-entry

refractoriness

regurgitant heart valve

serum enzymes

shunt

stenotic heart valve

sublingual

substernal

tachycardia

tamponade

tetralogy of Fallot

thrombolytic

transmural

variant angina

—Other teaching strategies

A. Have students use blood pressure measuring equipment to check for pulsus paradoxus.

B. If an electrocardiograph machine is available, do an electrocardiogram (ECG) and explain the tracing in terms of the P, Q, R, S, and T waves. You can also use the electrocardiograph to demonstrate the effect of respiratory movements on the autonomic nervous system control of heart rate. Have the student perform a 15 second Valsalva maneuver to alter preload (venous return decreases during the strain and heart rate should increase) and afterload (greater immediately following release of strain [about 4 to 7 heartbeats] when increased venous return is ejected into an arterial tree that remains constricted because of baroreceptor mechanisms that were induced during the strain). The poststrain blood pressure overshoot should produce a 1 to 2 cardiac cycle slowing of heart rate. Having the student perform maximal inspiration and expiration will demonstrate the normal variation in heart rate that occurs with respiration. This variation is called the respiratory sinus arrhythmia (RSA) and is thought to be a purely vagal response. The heart rate response to both the Valsalva maneuver and forced respiration should be more pronounced in a younger student (18 to 30 years).

C. Use ECG tracing obtained from a clinical setting to illustrate different types of dysrhythmias.

Chapter 24

Heart Failure

Chapter 24 focuses on heart failure irrespective of cause. It explains the manifestations of heart failure in terms of cardiac reserve and the compensatory mechanisms used to maintain the cardiac reserve. The hemodynamics of right-sided and left-sided heart failure are discussed separately. Right heart failure and left heart failure are discussed separately. The chapter ends with a discussion of heart transplant as a treatment method for some persons with end-stage heart disease.

Teaching strategies

—Overhead transparencies

Figure 24-3 shows the ejection fractions with normal heart function and with systolic and diastolic dysfunction.

Figures 24-4 and 24-5 compare the hemodynamic manifestations of right-sided and left-sided heart failure.

—Glossary terms

cardiac reserve

Frank-Starling mechanism

ascites

cardiac cachexia

cardiac glycosides

cyanosis

exertional dyspnea

orthopnea

nocturia

Cheyne-Stokes respirations

Swan-Ganz catheter

thermodilution measurement of cardiac output

—Other teaching strategies

A. Draw the Starling curve on the blackboard or on an overhead to demonstrate the effect of digitalis on cardiac output in a person with heart failure. Extend the Starling curve to include the descending limb and explain its significance in terms of cardiac output and cardiac reserve. Explain how the administration of diuretics could reduce vascular volume, left end-diastolic volume, and move a person with heart failure from the descending limb where cardiac output is decreased to the top or ascending limb of the Starling curve where cardiac output will be greater.

Chapter 25

Circulatory Shock

Circulatory shock represents failure of the circulatory system. It can be caused by failure of the heart as a pump (cardiogenic shock), by a disparity between the size of the vascular compartment and the amount of fluid that fills the compartment. This disparity can result from a loss in vascular volume (hypovolemic shock), an increase in the size of the compartment so that it is inadequately filled (distributive shock), or impeded flow through the central circulation (obstructive shock). Chapter 23 focuses on the types of shock, compensatory mechanisms, manifestations, complications, and treatment of shock.

Teaching strategies

—Overhead transparencies

Figure 25-1 compares the altered hemodynamic status that occurs with hypovolemic, cardiogenic, obstructive, and distributive shock.

—Glossary terms

aerobic and anaerobic metabolism

glycolysis

hemodynamic

nutrient and non-nutrient capillary flow

sensorium

shock (anaphylactic, cardiogenic, compensated, distributive, hypovolemic, neurogenic, obstructive) hemodynamic

vasodilator substances

vasoconstriction

Chapter 26

Control of Respiratory Function

Chapter 26 was designed to assist students in understanding the respiratory system and normal respiratory function. It is suggested that students read this chapter in preparation for understanding content in Chapters 25 and 26. The chapter is organized into 4 parts: (1) the structural organization of the respiratory system, (2) exchange of gases between the atmosphere and the lungs, (3) exchange and transport of gases in the body, and (4) control of respiration. The chapter includes a discussion of atmospheric and respiratory pressures, lung volumes and capacities obtained using the spirometer, ventilation-perfusion relationships including dead air space and shunt, the oxygen-dissociation curve and dissolved oxygen, carbon dioxide transport, control of breathing, and the cough reflex.

Teaching strategies

—Overhead transparencies

Figure 26-1 shows the structures of the respiratory system.

Figure 26-5 depicts a lobule of the lung, showing the bronchial smooth muscle fibers, pulmonary blood vessels, and lymphatics.

Figure 26-8 illustrates the movement of the respiratory muscles during inspiration and expiration.

Figure 26-11 illustrates surface tension in the alveoli and the role of surfactant in reducing surface tension.

Figure 26-12 illustrates the relationship between intrapleural pressure and airway pressure in terms of causing airway collapse during expiration.

Figure 26-14 shows the matching of ventilation and perfusion in the normally ventilated and perfused alveoli, in an alveoli that is perfused and not ventilated (shunt), and in an alveoli that is ventilated but not perfused (dead air space).

Figure 26-15 represents the oxygen dissociation curve.

—Glossary terms

airway resistance

alveoli (type 1 and type 2 alveolar cells)

antitussive

apnea

atmospheric pressure

bronchioles

bronchospasm

chemoreceptors

compliance

conducting airways

dead air space

diffusion

dyspnea

epiglottis

expectorate

expectorant

expiration

expiratory reserve volume

goblet cells

hypercapnia

hyperpnia

hyperventilation

hypoxia

inspiration

inspiratory reserve volume

intrapleural pressure

intrapulmonary pressure

intrathoracic pressure

larynx

mucociliary blanket

partial pressure

periodic breathing

pharynx

pleura

relative humidity

residual volume

respiratory tissues

spirometry

sputum

surface tension

surfactant

tidal volume

total lung volume

tracheobronchial tree

transpulmonary pressure

ventilation

viscid

vital capacity

water vapor pressure

—Other teaching strategies

Application of the law of LaPlace and inflation of small and large alveoli. This demonstration uses two new balloons of same size and from same manufacturer (the assumption being that the tension is the walls of new balloons is equal) and a plastic Y tube (3/8 to 1/2 inch diameter). Plug the base of the Y tube to prevent air from escaping. Blow up the two balloon—one with a small amount of air and the other with a larger amount. Twist the ends of the balloons as they are inflated to prevent air from escaping and insert one on each of the Y limbs of the Y tube. Now ask students which balloon they think should empty into which when the ends of the balloons are opened up and air is allow to flow freely between the two balloons. Untwist the balloons and observe the movement of air—from the smaller balloon which has the greater pressure to the larger balloon which has the lesser pressure. Movement of air follows the law of LaPlace (Figure 17-9): Pressure (P) = 2 Tension (2T)/radius of sphere or in this case alveoli (R) eg. 10 (P) = 20 (T)/2 (R) large balloon 20 (P) = 20 (T)/1 (R) small balloon. This demonstration can be used to emphasize: (1) the need for surfactant to decrease effort needed for inflation of the smaller alveoli, (2) the fact that the pressure needed to inflate the lung becomes less at higher lung volumes (pressure-volume curve), and (3) the need for deep breathing in post-operative and immobilized patients to maintain inflation of the small airways and alveoli and to prevent their collapse. This is because wall tension increases as the airway radius decreases and airway collapse occurs when wall tension exceeds inflation pressure (the critical closing pressure).

Chapter 27

Alterations in Respiratory Function

Chapter 27 focuses on alterations in respiratory function. The chapter is organized into six sections: respiratory tract infections, disorders of the pleura, obstructive lung disorders, interstitial lung diseases, pulmonary vascular disorders, and cancer of the lung. The section on respiratory infections includes the common cold and acute respiratory infections in children. Both Legionnaires' disease and pneumocystis pneumonia are included in this section as are the current recommendations for influenza and pneumococcal immunization. The sections on disorders of the pleura provides a description of pleural pain and how it can be differentiated from other types of pain.

Teaching strategies

—Overhead transparencies

Figure 27-1 compares the location of involvement in bronchopneumonia and lobar pneumonia.

Figure 27-3 illustrates the mechanisms of altered lung inflation in absorption and compression atelectasis.

Figure 27-7 illustrates the pathology in bronchiectasis.

—Glossary terms

asbestos	interstitial lung disease
asthma	lobar pneumonia
atelectasis	mucoviscidosis
blastomycosis	mycoplasmas
bronchial pneumonia	paraneoplastic
bronchiectasis	pleural effusion
bronchiolitis	pneumothorax
chylothorax	pulmonary embolism
coccidiomycosis	sarcoidosis
cor pulmonale	silicosis
croup	sternal retraction
decongestant	stridor
emphysema	thoracentesis
empyema	tubercle
epiglottitis	wheezing
hemothorax	
histoplasmosis	

—Other teaching strategies

A. Lung compliance and ease of lung inflation. Use two balloons to demonstrate effect of lung compliance (Compliance = Volume/pressure) on lung inflation. Inflate one balloon and allow to remain inflated overnight (this will decrease the elasticity of the rubber and make the balloon more compliant) and leave the other balloon uninflated (this balloon will be less complaint than the inflated balloon). During class the instructor can demonstrate the effort (similar to breathing effort) needed to inflate the compliant and noncompliant balloons. The noncompliant balloon can be compared to a lung with restrictive lung disease, pulmonary edema, or adult respiratory disease. The complaint balloon is similar to the emphysematous lung.

Chapter 28

Alterations in Control of Ventilation and Respiratory Failure

Chapter 28 describes alterations in control of ventilation and respiratory failure. The chapter incorporates a discussion of drug induced respiratory depression and weakness of the respiratory muscles, sleep apnea, sudden infant death syndrome, hyperventilation syndrome, and acute respiratory failure.

Teaching strategies

—Glossary terms

adult respiratory distress syndrome (ARDS)	central and obstructive sleep apnea
carbon dioxide narcosis	hyaline membrane
	REM sleep

Examination questions

1. The red blood cell has a life span of approximately:

   a. 30 days
   b. 60 days
   ● c. 120 days
   d. 360 days

2. The process of conjugation:

   a. breaks hemoglobin into bilirubin, globulin chains, and iron
   b. generates the intermediate 2,3-diphosphoglycerate (2,3-DPG) functions in controlling the affinity of hemoglobin for oxygen
   c. acts to maintain hemoglobin in the reduced state so that it can function in oxygen transport
   ● d. renders lipid soluble bilirubin from senescent red into a water soluble form.

3. The hematocrit measures:

   a. the number of red blood cells
   b. the hemoglobin content of blood
   ● c. the percentage of red cells in a given volume of blood
   d. the size of the red blood cells

4. Anemia is most accurately defined as:

   a. hemorrhage
   ● b. low numbers of red blood cells and/or hemoglobin
   c. red cell hemolysis
   d. an iron deficiency state

5. Which one of the following conditions can lead to the development of hemolytic anemia:

   ● a. transfusion reaction
   b. hemorrhage
   c. bone marrow depression
   d. dietary deficiency of iron

6. The cause of pernicious anemia is:

   a. the absence of extrinsic factor
   ● b. the absence of intrinsic factor
   c. lack of vitamin B 12 in the diet
   d. iron deficiency

7. Conditions which predispose to sickling of hemoglobin in persons with sickle cell anemia are those that:

   a. impair red blood cell maturation
   b. increase the iron content of blood
   c. increase the oxygen content of the blood
   ● d. increase the level of deoxygenated hemoglobin

8. Iron deficiency anemia is most common in:

   ● a. infants, adolescents, and pregnant women
   b. middle-aged men and women
   c. young and middle-aged men
   d. older men and women

9. Signs and symptoms of anemia correspond most closely with those associated with:

   a. iron deficiency
   b. hypovolemia
   • c. hypoxia
   d. hypotension

10. An individual with polycythemia might be expected to have:

   • a. increased red blood cells and increased blood pressure
   b. increased red blood cells and decreased blood volume
   c. decreased red blood cells and increased blood pressure
   d. decreased red blood cells and decreased blood pressure

11. Which type of ABO antibodies would a person with type O blood have?:

   a. A
   • b. AB
   c. B
   d. O

12. Which part of the circulatory system contain the greatest amount of blood:

   a. the systemic arteries
   • b. the systemic veins
   c. the systemic capillaries
   d. the pulmonary arteries and veins

13. Which one of the following exerts the greatest effect on blood flow:

   • a. vessel radius
   b. vessel length
   c. change in blood pressure
   d. blood viscosity

14. Peripheral vascular resistance can best be defined as:

   a. constriction of the blood vessels in the circulatory system
   • b. blood pressure needed to overcome the resistance to flow in the circulatory system
   c. frictional forces in the circulatory system
   d. the sum of vessel constriction and blood viscosity

15. A reduction in the cross-sectional area of a blood vessel will produce:

   a. a decrease in velocity of blood flow
   • b. an increase in velocity of blood flow
   c. an increase in potential energy and stretching of the vessel wall
   d. a decreased potential for development of turbulent flow

16. According to the law of Laplace, the reason that small blood vessels collapse during circulatory shock is that the:

   a. wall tension needed to maintain vessel patency is reduced due to a fall in blood pressure
   b. wall tension is decreased due to a decrease in blood volume and vessel radius
   • c. blood pressure drops to a point where it can no longer overcome the increased tension in the vessel wall resulting from a decrease in blood volume and vessel radius

17. In which segment of the arterial system would you normally expect to find the greatest pulse pressure:

   a. the aorta
   b. the brachial artery
   c. the femoral artery
   • d. the dorsalis pedis

18. Which one of the following statements is true as it relates to the venous system. Veins:

- a. are thin walled vessels that function in storage of blood
  b. lack innervation by the sympathetic nervous system
  c. have high intraluminal pressures
  d. are not influenced by the effects of gravity

19. Autoregulation of blood flow in the microcirculation is primarily controlled by:

- a. the metabolic needs of the tissues
  b. the blood pressure
  c. autonomic nervous system
  d. cardiac output

20. Redness which follows temporary occlusion of superficial blood vessels is due to:

  a. development of collateral circulation
  b. venous congestion
- c. hyperemia associated with a compensatory increase in capillary flow
  d. vessel engorgement resulting from inflammation

21. An embolus can be described as:

  a. a blood clot in the arterial system
  b. an obstruction of blood flow due to the presence of a blood clot
- c. a foreign mass that is transported in the blood stream
  d. a moving blood clot

22. Atherosclerosis affects:

- a. large and medium sized arteries
  b. small arteries
  c. veins
  d. vessels of the microcirculation

23. According to the American Heart Association, major risk factors for atherosclerosis that can be changed include:

- a. hypertension, cigarette smoking, blood cholesterol levels
  b. heredity, female sex, cigarette smoking
  c. physical inactivity, male sex, blood cholesterol levels
  d. Stress, hypertension, smoking, high density lipoprotein levels

24. Which one of the following lipoproteins is the major carrier of cholesterol:

  a. chylomicrons
  b. VLDLs
- c. LDLs
  d. HDLs

25. The receptors that bind and remove LDL carrying cholesterol from the circulation are mainly located in the:

  a. blood vessels
- b. liver
  c. spleen
  d. kidney

26. Dietary factors that increase serum cholesterol and its lipoprotein fraction are:

  a. excess alcohol intake, insoluble fiber, and simple sugars
  b. excess calories, saturated fats, cholesterol
  c. lack of vitamin C, saturated fats, cholesterol
- d. complex carbohydrates, saturated fats, cholesterol

27. A dissecting aneurysm can be described as:

  a. an outpouching of a major arterial vessel
  b. a tortuous defect in a vein
  c. multiple small dilatations of an artery
- d. separation and bleeding between the layers of an arterial wall.

28. Because of its arterial location, often the first sign of an abdominal aneurysm is:

● a. a pulsating abdominal mass
   b. an enlarged liver
   c. complaints of abdominal or back pain
   d. constipation

29. Raynaud's phenomenon is caused by:

● a. spasm of arterial vessels
   b. inflammatory changes of the artery
   c. atherosclerosis
   d. thrombosis due to venous insufficiency

30. Which of the following observations suggest the presence of peripheral vascular disease of the lower extremity:

● a. complaints of pain on walking which are relieved by rest
   b. thickened skin over the feet and ankle area
   c. legs become pale when in the dependent position and reddened when elevated
   d. sensation of increased pulsations in the popliteal and pedal arteries

31. Two factors that predispose to the development of varicose veins are:

● a. obesity and standing for long periods of time
   b. weight loss and increased use of the skeletal muscle pumps
   c. immobility and aging
   d. menopause and hypertension

32. Conditions which contribute to the development of venous thrombosis include:

● a. immobility
   b. hypertension
   c. a decrease in level of coagulation factors
   d. weight loss

33. One of the most important manifestations of the compartment syndrome is:

● a. unrelenting pain that is greater than expected for the primary condition
   b. absent pulses and abnormal capillary refill time
   c. pallor of the affected extremity
   d. lack of neurologic manifestations

34. Tissue injury due to shearing forces occurs when:

   a. blood flow is occluded as a result of tissue pressure
● b. blood flow is occluded due to stretching and angulation of blood vessels as one tissue layer slides over another
   c. sliding movements cause removal of the outer skin layers
   d. heat is generated as the result of frictional forces that develop as one tissue layer slides over another

35. Which stage pressure ulcer is characterized by partial- thickness skin loss involving the epidermis or dermis, or both:

   a. stage I
● b. stage II
   c. stage III
   d. stage IV

36. The systolic blood pressure reflects the:

● a. stroke volume output and the distensibility of the aorta
   b. heart rate and the resistance to flow encountered in the arterioles
   c. the competency of the aortic valve and resistance to flow encountered in the arterioles
   d. The difference between the highest and lowest points on the pressure tracing

37. The sympathetic nervous system regulates blood pressure through its effect on:

   ● a. heart rate, strength of myocardial contraction, and peripheral vascular resistance
   b. blood vessel tone and indirectly through its effect on anxiety levels
   c. vascular volume
   d. angiotensin and aldosterone levels

38. Long-term regulation of blood pressure depends on function of the:

   a. arterial baroreceptors
   b. chemoreceptors
   c. autonomic nervous system
   ● d. kidneys in terms of regulating body levels of salt and water

39. Factors that predispose to the development of essential hypertension include:

   ● a. obesity and high sodium intake
   b. coarctation of the aorta and kidney disease
   c. atherosclerosis and pregnancy
   d. brain ischemia and excess adrenal cortical hormone levels

40. Preeclampsia is characterized by:

   a. exaggeration of pre-existing hypertension that occurs during pregnancy
   b. hypertension that is noted before the 20th week of pregnancy
   ● c. hypertension of pregnancy, weight gain in excess of 2 pounds/week, and proteinuria
   d. hypertension that persists after pregnancy

41. Isolated systolic hypertension in the elderly can best be explained in terms of:

   a. increased salt retention that occurs with aging
   b. increased baroreceptor function that occurs with aging
   ● c. increased rigidity of the aorta that occurs with aging
   d. increased blood viscosity that occurs with aging

42. The auscultatory gap which occurs in some elderly persons can lead to:

   ● a. underestimation of systolic blood pressure
   b. overestimation of systolic blood pressure
   c. underestimation of diastolic blood pressure
   d. overestimation of diastolic blood pressure

43. Blood pressure readings in persons with a pheochromocytoma are usually highest:

   a. during sleep
   b. in the standing position
   c. in the supine position
   ● d. during periods of stress

44. Limiting salt intake is recommended as an initial nonpharmacological treatment for hypertension because it:

   a. helps a person lose weight
   ● b. reduces water retention and decreases vascular volume
   c. reduces sympathetic nervous system activity
   d. increases cardiac output and reduces renal blood flow

45. When used in the treatment of hypertension, a₁-adrenergic blockers reduce the effect of the sympathetic nervous system on:

    a. heart rate
    b. cardiac output
    c. renin release
    • d. vascular smooth muscle tone

46. The most common cause of skeletal muscle pump weakness, decreased venoconstrictor tone, and reduced blood volume that predispose to orthostatic hypotension is:

    a. fluid deficit
    b. old age
    c. impaired autonomic nervous system function
    • d. bed rest

47. The function of the heart valves is to:

    a. control the rate at which blood moves through the heart
    b. regulate the flow of electrical activity between the atria and ventricles of the heart
    • c. provide for unidirectional flow of blood through the heart
    d. control the inflow of blood into the atria

48. The order of impulse conduction in the heart is from the:

    a. AV node to SA node to bundle of His to Purkinje system
    b. bundle of His to SA node to AV node to Purkinje system
    • c. SA node to AV node to bundle of His to Purkinje system
    d. Purkinje system to SA node to AV node to bundle of His

49. Phase 2 of a cardiac muscle action potential represents:

    a. depolarization
    b. repolarization
    • c. the plateau
    d. resting membrane potential

50. Sympathetic stimulation of the heart will:

    • a. increase heart rate and increase the strength of cardiac contraction
    b. constrict coronary blood vessels and decrease the metabolic activity of the heart
    c. increase heart rate and decrease the strength of myocardial contraction
    d. decrease heart rate and increase the metabolic activity of the heart

51. According to Starling's law of the heart:

    • a. increasing venous return produces an increase in stroke volume output due to diastolic stretching of myocardial fibers
    b. increasing venous return produces an increase in cardiac output via sympathetic nervous system mechanisms
    c. increased cardiac output results from increased cardiac contractility that is unrelated to the resting muscle length
    d. increasing the force against which the heart must pump increases the pumping efficiency of the heart

52. The reason that coronary blood flow is less during systole than during diastole is because:

    a. the duration of systole is shorter than diastole
    b. the atrioventricular valves are closed during systole
    c. the diastolic pressure is less during systole
    • d. the contracting myocardial fibers compress the intramyocardial blood vessels during systole

53. With an increase in heart rate, stroke volume will decrease because of:

   a. increased blood pressure and total peripheral resistance
 • b. decreased diastolic filling time
   c. decreased systolic ejection time
   d. decreased coronary perfusion and contractile strength

54. The main preload work of the heart results from:

 • a. venous return to the heart
   b. the arterial blood pressure
   c. resistance to flow through the aortic valve
   d. the venous pressure

55. Which one of the following conditions would be expected to produce the greatest increase in heart work:

 • a. increased arterial blood pressure and stroke volume output
   b. decreased heart rate and increased stroke volume output
   c. decreased arterial blood pressure and heart rate
   d. decreased stroke volume output and decreased arterial blood pressure

56. Cardiac tamponade refers to:

 • a. an acute inflammation of the pericardial sac
   b. blocking of conduction through the atrioventricular node
   c. compression of the heart due to excess fluid in the pericardial sac
   d. an abnormal opening in the atrial septum of the heart

57. Pulsus paradoxus refers to:

   a. an irregular pulse
   b. a pulse rate that changes with the respiratory cycle
 • c. an exaggerated inspiratory decrease in systolic blood pressure
   d. presence of skipped heart beats

58. One of the reasons that persons with atherosclerotic heart disease do not usually experience pain until the vessel is largely occluded is because:

   a. collateral channels do not open until the coronary vessels are almost fully occluded
   b. the blood in the coronary vessels carries a large oxygen reserve to protect against reduced flow
   c. the threshold for activation of the pain fibers associated with the coronary blood vessels does not occur until they are fully compressed by the atherosclerotic process
 • d. blood flow is directly related to the fourth power of the vessel radius

59. The functional cause of angina is:

   a. atherosclerosis
   b. valvular heart disease
   c. congestive heart failure
 • d. disparity between oxygen supplied by the coronary vessels and the metabolic demands of the heart

60. Angina due to spasm of a coronary blood vessel is often referred to as:

   a. classical angina
 • b. variant (Prinzmetal's) angina
   c. unstable angina
   d. silent angina

61. Rest is beneficial in relieving the pain associated with angina because during rest:

   a. the coronary blood vessels dilate
   b. venous return to the heart is increased in the seated or supine position
   c. coronary blood flow is improved due to an increase in blood pressure
 • d. the coronary circulation is adequate to meet the metabolic needs of the heart

62. The signs and symptoms of myocardial infarction include:

    a. chest pain that is affected by breathing and is relieved by nitroglycerin
    • b. severe crushing chest pain and sensation of nausea and indigestion
    c. anxiety and chest pain that is affected by movement
    d. pain in the left arm that occurs on arising and is accompanied by tingling and weakness in the hand

63. The most common complication of early myocardial infarction is:

    a. congestive heart failure
    • b. dysrhythmias
    c. cardiogenic shock
    d. rupture of the heart

64. Following a heart attack, the myocardial tissue that has been replaced by scar tissue will:

    a. be able to contract
    • b. serve to maintain the continuity of myocardium
    c. be able to conduct impulses
    d. serve to maintain its elastic properties of the myocardial muscle fibers

65. In the normal electrocardiogram (lead II):

    • a. a P wave precedes every QRS complex, the P-R interval is less than .21 seconds, and both the QRS and T wave are positive deflections
    b. a P wave precedes every QRS complex, the P-R interval is greater than .21 seconds, the QRS is a positive deflection, and the T wave is negative deflection
    c. a P wave precedes every second or third QRS complex, and the QRS and T wave are positive
    d. a P wave precedes every QRS complex, the QRS complex is greater than .21 seconds, and the T wave is positive

66. The term ectopic pacemaker describes:

    • a. an excitable focus outside the normal conduction system
    b. an excitable focus within the normal conduction system
    c. scar tissue that forms a block to the conduction of cardiac impulses
    d. an area of the heart that is refractory to normal conduction of cardiac impulses

67. In complete A-V nodal block (third-degree block):

    a. there is a prolongation of the P-R interval
    • b. the atria and ventricles beat independently of each other
    c. there is a failure in conduction of every second or third impulse from the atria to the ventricles

68. Dilated cardiomyopathy exerts its greatest effect through:

    a. production of dysrhythmias
    b. hypertrophy of the left ventricle
    c. reduced filling of the heart
    • d. decreased stroke volume output

69. Rheumatic fever is essentially a preventable form of heart disease that results from:

    a. direct invasion of heart tissue by group-A hemolytic streptococcus
    • b. an immune response which involves the group-A hemolytic streptococcus
    c. a viral infection of the heart
    d. the presence of group-a hemolytic streptococcus toxins

70. The most common cause of acute infective endocarditis is:

    rheumatic fever
    • intravenous drug abuse
    intravenous catheters that used in hospitals
    prosthetic heart valves

71. The predisposing factors associated with development of subacute infective endocarditis are:

    a. reduced resistance of the host and a bacterial infection

    b. a severe infection and coronary heart disease

 • c. a portal of entry for the microorganism and a damaged endocardium

    d. presence of antibodies for the offending organism and reduced host resistance

72. With advanced mitral stenosis, there is:

 • a. increased pressure in the pulmonary veins and pulmonary edema

    b. systolic heart murmur and hypertrophy of the left ventricle

    c. increased stroke volume output from the left ventricle and an exaggerated pulse pressure

    d. decreased pulmonary blood flow and cyanosis

73. Cor pulmonale describes:

 • a. congestive right-sided heart failure due to long standing pulmonary hypertension

    b. an associated congenital heart and lung disorder

    c. pulmonary congestion due to left-sided heart failure

    d. stenosis of the pulmonary valve

74. In atrial septal defects, pulmonary hypertension is most directly related to:

 • a. increased blood flow through the pulmonary vessels

    b. premature maturation of the pulmonary blood vessels

    c. increased viscosity of blood due to a compensatory polycythemia

    d. increased resistance to outflow of blood from the left heart

75. Congenital heart disease involving a left-to-right shunt is generally characterized by which of the following:

    a. movement of unoxygenated blood into the systemic circulation and cyanosis

 • b. increased pulmonary blood flow and risk of pulmonary hypertension

    c. increased ejection of blood from the left ventricle and risk of systemic hypertension

    d. increased pulmonary blood flow due to increased venous return to the heart

76. In Tetralogy of Fallot there is:

    a. right atrial and left atrial hypertrophy, interatrial and interventricular septal defects

 • b. right ventricular hypertrophy, stenosis of the pulmonary artery, ventricular septal defect with displacement of the aorta so that it overrides the defect

    c. persistence of the embryonic vessel connecting the pulmonary artery to the descending aorta with hypertrophy of the left ventricle

    d. origination of the aorta from the right ventricle and origination of the pulmonary artery from the left ventricle

77. Congestive heart failure can best be described as:

    a. excessive hypertrophy of the heart

 • b. inability of the heart to pump sufficient blood to meet the needs of the body

    c. condition that develops because of coronary heart disease

    d. impaired pumping ability due to cardiac dysrhythmias

78. The cardiac reserve refers to:

    a. the ability of the coronary vessels to supply blood to the myocardium

    b. the ability of the heart to increase its rate

 • c. the maximum percentage of increase in cardiac output (as compared to resting output) that can be achieved

79. Signs and symptoms of heart failure are most directly related to:

    a. cardiac distention
    b. cardiac hypertrophy
    • c. impaired pumping ability of the heart
    d. dysrhythmias

80. In heart failure, dyspnea often develops when the person has been lying down for several hours. This is because assumption of the the supine position causes:

    a. decreased blood return to the right heart
    b. an increase in arterial pressure
    • c. mobilization and redistribution of edema fluid from the dependent areas of the body to the lungs

81. Signs and symptoms of left-sided heart failure include:

    • a. cyanosis, cough with frothy sputum, fine pulmonary rales
    b. edema of the dependent extremities and orthopnea
    c. enlargement of the liver and anorexia
    d. cyanosis and peripheral edema

82. Circulatory shock can best be described as a condition in which there is:

    a. a state of hypotension
    b. loss of blood
    c. loss of consciousness due to blood loss
    • d. inadequate blood flow to meet the metabolic needs of body tissues

83. In shock one of the best indicators of blood flow to vital organs is:

    a. rate of blood and fluid administration
    b. blood pressure
    c. the color and temperature of the skin
    • d. urine output

84. Causes of hypovolemic shock include:

    • a. vomiting and loss of body fluids
    b. allergic reactions to drugs
    c. cardiac failure
    d. hypoglycemia

85. Early signs of hypovolemic shock include:

    • a. restlessness, thirst, and increased heart rate
    b. decreased blood pressure and apathy
    c. increase in heart rate and increased pulse pressure
    d. decreased blood pressure and unconsciousness

86. The pale, cool, and "clammy" skin that is often observed in an individual with shock can best be explained in terms of:

    a. loss of red blood cells
    • b. body's attempt to shunt blood to vital organs by constricting skin vessels
    c. decreased metabolic needs that accompany shock
    d. body's attempt to conserve heat loss

87. Anaphylactic shock is associated with:

    • a. presence of vasodilator substances in the blood.
    b. failure of the heart as a pump
    c. loss of blood volume
    d. impaired activity of the vasomotor control centers

88. The gas exchange portion of the respiratory system consists of the:

    a. larynx and trachea
    b. bronchioles and alveoli
    • c. alveolar structures and pulmonary capillaries
    d. bronchi and broncioles

89. The moisture content of the air that is in the lung:

    a. is the same as that in the atmosphere
    b. is less than atmospheric
 • c. is maintained at a 100% relative humidity
    d. decreases as body temperature increases

90. The intrapleural pressure is normally negative in relation to:

    a. atmospheric pressure
 • b. intrapulmonary pressure

91. The main muscles of inspiration are the:

    a. intercostal muscles
 • b. diaphragm muscles
    c. accessory muscles
    d. abdominal muscles

92. Lung compliance refers to the ease with which:

 • a. the lungs can be inflated or the amount of pressure needed to change their volume
    b. air can be moved through the airway
    c. air can be exhaled from the lungs
    d. sputum can be expectorated from the lungs

93. Surface tension describes the:

 • a. forces that develop at the liquid air interface in the alveoli
    b. resistance to airflow in the small airways
    c. the elastic forces in the wall of the alveoli
    d. pressure in the pleural cavity

94. The minute volume (tidal volume respiratory rate) describes the amount of air that is exchanged (ventilated) in a minute. In restrictive lung disease, the:

 • a. respiratory rate is increased and the tidal volume is decreased
    b. respiratory rate is decreased and the tidal volume increased
    c. both respiratory rate and tidal volume are increased
    d. both the respiratory rate and tidal volume are decreased

95. The term vital capacity refers to:

    a. the amount of air taken in and exhaled during normal respiration
 • b. maximal amount of air that can be taken in and exhaled with forceful expiration
    c. the amount of air that remains in the lung after forceful expiration
    d. the amount of air that can be forcefully exhaled after normal inspiration

96. An anatomic shunt is one in which:

 • a. blood moves directly from the venous to the arterial side of the circulation without moving through the lungs
    b. blood moves through an unventilated portion of the lungs
    c. air moves into an unperfused area of the lung
    d. neither neither air nor blood moves into an area of the lung

97. In which one of the following situations would the diffusing capacity of the lung be impaired because of a decrease in surface area:

    a. pneumonia
 • b. surgical removal of a lung
    c. pulmonary edema
    d. anemia

98. Most of the oxygen carried in the blood is transported:

   a. in the dissolved form in the plasma
 • b. attached to hemoglobin

99. The PO2 levels of the blood refer to the oxygen that is:

 • a. dissolved in the plasma
   b. attached to the hemoglobin molecules of the red blood cells

100. Most of the carbon dioxide that is produced as a result of tissue metabolism is carried in the blood in the form of:

   a. dissolved carbon dioxide
   b. carboxihemoglobin
 • c. bicarbonate

101. Which one of the following would differentiate acute from chronic hypoxia:

 • a. polycythemia
   b. dyspnea
   c. fatigue
   d. cyanosis

102. Conditions that impair closure of the glottis such as the presence of a nasogastric tube impair coughing by:

   a. suppressing the innervation of the respiratory muscles needed for coughing
   b. impairing inspiration and full lung expansion
 • c. preventing the full increase in intrathoracic pressure needed for an effective cough
   d. increasing the viscosity of respiratory tract secretions

103. The most common vehicle for transmission of the common cold is:

   a. air droplets which contain the virus
   b. contaminated dishes and silverware
 • c. the fingers
   d. contaminated towels and facial tissues

104. A distinguishing feature of influenza is:

   a. dry and nonproductive cough
 • b. abrupt onset symptoms of fever, chills, and general malaise
   c. fever and headache
   d. sore throat and profuse water nasal discharge

105. Bronchopneumonia is characterized by:

   a. involvement of a large portion or lobe of a lung
 • b. patchy consolidation of lung tissue with involvement of multiple lobes
   c. inflammation that is confined to the interstitial tissue that surrounds the alveoli and bronchioles
   d. inflammation of the larger airways

106. Compared to lobar pneumonia, bronchopneumonia:

   a. has a sudden onset with shaking chills and fever
 • b. has an insidious onset and greater incidence of complications
   c. is only caused by the Streptococcus pneumoniae
   d. only affects young or otherwise healthy persons

107. The lesions associated with tuberculosis are caused by:

 • a. immune mechanisms
   b. the destructive nature of the tubercle baccilus
   c. enzymes released from the tubercle baccilus
   d. the entrance of the tubercle baccilus into lung cells

108. A positive tuberculin skin indicates that:

   a. an individual has tuberculosis
   b. an individual has never been exposed to tuberculosis
 • c. an individual has been exposed and sensitized to the tubercle baccilus
   d. is susceptible to developing tuberculosis

109. Which one of the fungal infections of the lung is spread through bird excreta:

- a. histoplasmosis
  b. coccidioidomycosis
  c. blastomycosis

110. Pleural pain is usually:

- a. unilateral and is made worse by chest movements
  b. substernal and radiates to the shoulder or arm
  c. bilateral and located in the inferior portions of the chest cage
  d. substernal and dull in character

111. In tension pneumothorax, you would expect signs and symptoms to arise because intrathoracic pressure becomes:

- a. greater than atmospheric
  b. less than atmospheric
  c. equal to atmospheric

112. Which of the following signs and symptoms is suggestive of a tension pneumothorax (with mediastinal shift) as compared to an open pneumothorax in which air moves freely into and out of the chest:

  a. dyspnea
  b. lack of chest expansion during inspiration
  c. absence of breath sounds
- d. deviation of the trachea

113. Atelectasis refers to:

  a. collapse of an entire lung
  b. fluid in the pleural space
  c. inflammation of the pleura
- d. incomplete expansion of a portion of the lung

114. Which one of the following is most descriptive of the signs and symptoms of atelectasis:

- a. dyspnea, increased respiratory rate, and absence of breath sounds and presence of intercostal retractions over the involved area
  b. dyspnea, decreased respiratory rate, and presence of rales over the affected area
  c. dyspnea, productive cough, rhonchi, and use of the accessory muscles for breathing
  d. dyspnea, cyanosis, and presence of rales over the affected area

115. Increased parasympathetic activity causes:

- a. constriction of the bronchioles
  b. relaxation of the bronchioles

116. In bronchial asthma, the early response involves:

- a. an antigen-antibody response
  b. inflammation and increased airway responsiveness

117. During an asthmatic attack:

- a. the residual lung volume is increased and vital capacity decreased
  b. the inspiratory reserve volume is decreased and vital capacity increased
  c. the residual volume is decreased and vital capacity increased
  d. the inspiratory reserve volume is increased and vital capacity decreased

118. In chronic obstructive pulmonary disease (COPD) there is:

  a. Obstruction of the trachea and larynx
- b. small airway obstruction during the expiratory phase of ventilation
  c. obstructed airflow in the bronchi during inspiration
  d. airway obstruction due to collapse of portions of the lung

119. Persons with COPD have a decrease in their $FEV_{1.0}$ that is measured during pulmonary function studies. The $FEV_{1.0}$ refers to:

   a. the amount of air that can be exchanged during normal breathing

 ● b. the maximal amount of air that is exhaled in one second

   c. the maximal amount of air that can be exhaled after maximal inspiration

   d. the total volume of air that is contained in the lungs

120. In the person with COPD, pursed-lip breathing improves ventilation because it:

   a. increases intraabdominal pressure as a means of facilitating descent of the diaphragm

 ● b. increases small airway pressures during expiration as a means of preventing their collapse

   c. increases vital capacity

   d. improves airflow by changing the position of the trachea

121. In persons with COPD the use of abdominal breathing training:

 ● a. produces relaxation and is used to reduce stress

   b. improves abdominal muscle tone and is used to increase respiratory rate

   c. reduces intra-abdominal pressure and allows for fuller descent of the diaphragm during inspiration

   d. prevents constipation and abdominal distention from occurring

122. The administration of continuous (18 - 24 hours/day) low-flow oxygen to a person with COPD who have a low PO_2 is beneficial because it:

 ● a. decreases the stimulus for pulmonary hypertension and polycythemia,

   b. increases the red blood cells and activity tolerance

   c. improves ventilation and decreases PCO_2 levels

   d. increases respiratory rate and gas exchange

123. Administering of high concentrations of oxygen to a person with chronic hypoxia can be harmful because:

   a. high concentrations are irritating to mucous membranes

 ● b. high concentrations suppress the oxygen chemoreceptors which provide the main stimulus for ventilation

   c. in high concentrations, the viscosity of oxygen increases airway resistance

   d. high concentrations of oxygen can cause bronchospasm

124. With upper airway obstruction in the infant and small child, retraction of chest structures occurs because:

   a. the lungs of a child are smaller than those of an adult

   b. mouth breathing is more common in children

 ● c. cartilaginous support in large airways has not been fully developed in the child

   d. children have a more rapid respiratory rate than adults

125. Which one of the following acute respiratory infections in children poses the greatest threat of severe hypoxia due to airway obstruction:

   a. the common cold

   b. bronchiolitis

   c. croup

 ● d. epiglottitis

126. Which one of the following could cause hypoxemia but not cyanosis:

    a. congestive heart failure
    b. chronic obstructive lung disease
 • c. anemia
    d. pneumonia

127. Cheyne-Stokes respirations can best be described as:

    a. rapid shallow respirations with increased length of the expiratory phase
    b. regular rhythmic respirations with periods of apnea
 • c. waxing and waning of respirations with periods of apnea
    d. labored breathing

128. The term dyspnea implies:

    a. a condition of labored breathing
    b. inability to breath easily when lying down
 • c. subjective complaints of breathlessness or difficult breathing
    d. irregular breathing

129. An early manifestation of sleep apnea is:

    a. rapid breathing during sleep
    b. periodic breathing during sleep
    c. shallow breathing during sleep
 • d. noisy snoring during sleep

130. Hyperventilation refers to:

    a. rapid breathing
    b. rapid irregular breathing
    c. rapid shallow breathing
 • d. excessive ventilation as indicated by a decrease in blood carbon dioxide levels

131. The breathing muscles that are usually used by persons with hyperventilation are the:

    a. diaphragm muscles
    b. abdominal muscles
 • c. intercostal and accessory muscles

132. Causes of respiratory failure due to impaired gas diffusion include:

    a. upper airway obstruction
    b. pulmonary embolism
    c. drug overdose
 • d. adult respiratory distress syndrome

133. Which of the following arterial blood gas levels would be suggestive of respiratory failure:

    a. PO_2 70 mm Hg and PCO_2 60 mm Hg
    b. PO_2 60 mm Hg and PCO_2 50 mm Hg
    c. PO_2 50 mm Hg and PCO_2 45 mm Hg
 • d. PO_2 45 mm Hg and PCO_2 60 mm Hg

134. Signs of hypercapnia include:

 • a. headache, flushed skin, and conjunctival hyperemia
    b. difficulty in problem solving and impaired vision
    c. confusion, tachycardia, and cyanosis
    d. Euphoria, confusion, and cyanosis

135. In persons with adult respiratory distress syndrome:

 • a. diffusion is impaired and the lungs become stiff and difficult to inflate
    b. there is air-trapping and difficulty in the expiration phase of ventilation
    c. portions of the lung collapse decreasing the area for gas diffusion
    d. there is loss of lung elasticity and mismatching of ventilation and perfusion

Alterations in Body Fluids

Fluids are essential components of a biological system; they vary in amount and composition, according to their location and purpose. The composition of body fluids is largely determined by the kidneys which filter the blood and eliminate those materials that are needed to maintain the constancy of the internal environment. This unit has been divided into six chapters: (1) alterations in body fluids and electrolytes, (2) alterations in distribution of body fluids: edema, (3) alterations in acid-base balance, (4) control of renal function, (5) alterations in renal function, and (6) renal failure.

Chapter 29

Alterations in Body Fluids and Electrolytes

Chapter 29 focuses on the composition and distribution of water and electrolytes in the intra- and extracellular fluid compartments. The chapter is organized into 4 parts: physiology of body composition and distribution, alterations in fluid volume, alterations in electrolyte composition of body fluids, and alterations in interstitial fluids and edema. The content on water and electrolytes is presented within a framework that considers: (1) the purpose or function of water or a given electrolyte, (2) body requirements including those related to age differences, (3) sources of gain and loss, and (4) body mechanisms for regulating water and electrolyte levels. Because of their impact on fluid and electrolyte balance, a discussion of thirst and thirst disorders; antidiuretic hormone (ADH) and disorders of ADH; and aldosterone are included in this chapter.

Teaching strategies

—Glossary terms

aldosterone

antidiuretic hormone (ADH)

capillary pressure

colloidal osmotic pressure

diabetes insipidus

diuresis

edema

electrolytes

extracellular

hydrostatic pressure

hyper and hypocalcemia

hyper and hypokalemia

hyper and hyponatremia

hypertonic

hypo- and hypermagnesmia

hypo- and hyperphosphatemia

hypotonic

insensible water losses

interstitial

intracellular

ion

isotonic

milliequivalent

milliosmol

mineralocorticoid   osmosis

nonelectrolytes   polydipsia

obligatory urine loss   polyuria

osmolality   tissue turgor

osmolarity   vasopressin

—Other teaching strategies

A. Have students calculate their electrolyte intake for one day using their nutrition textbook.

B. Have students examine the electrolyte content of various beverages, foods, salt substitute, and drugs.

C. Have student obtain the weight of a pint of water ('a pints a pound the world around') as a means of demonstrating that weight is an effective method for assessing the gain or loss of body water. Have students weigh a diaper before and after it is soaked with a given amount of water. Use a cold mirror to demonstrate insensible losses of water through breathing.

D. Provide laboratory values in a case study for persons with normal and altered electrolyte values. Have students explain possible altered body function.

E. Use the Nernst equation (Chapter 1) to explain the effects of altered serum sodium and potassium levels on the membrane potentials of excitable tissues and their possible consequences in terms of neuromuscular activity. This can be developed as a computer program for students to use.

F. Use a sponge to simulate the function of the tissue gel in the distribution of interstitial fluid and the development of pitting edema. When the sponge has been completely saturated with water, application of pressure causes water to move out of the sponge. If the sponge is on a table top, the water will move out onto its surface. This is similar to the mobile characteristics of water in tissues where the tissue gel has become fully saturated with water. Like tissue gel, water cannot be expressed from a sponge that is only slightly moistened. Unlike tissue gel, the sponge retains its shape and does not form an indentation when it is completely saturated and water is translocated.

Chapter 30

Alterations in Acid-Base Balance

Chapter 30 focuses on alterations in acid-base balance. The chapter is divided into two parts: the first part focuses on determination of pH and regulation of acid-base balance, while the second part covers alterations in acid-base balance

Teaching strategies

—Glossary terms

acid   alkalemia

acidemia   alkali

acidosis   alkalosis

anion gap   ketoacids

base excess and   ketosis
 deficit
                       lactic acidosis
buffer system
                       postprandial
carbonic anhydrase   alkaline tide

—Other teaching strategies

A. Have students use the Henderson-Hasselbalch equation to calculate pH with various pCO_2 and bicarbonate levels.

Chapter 31

Control of Renal Function

Chapter 31 reviews the structure and function of the kidneys. The statement from Homer W. Smith that is cited on p. 532 eloquently expresses the function of the kidneys in relation to the composition of body fluids. This chapter includes a discussion of tests of renal function and the action of diuretics.

Teaching strategies

—Overhead transparencies

Figure 31-2 shows the internal structures of the kidney.

Figure 31-3 shows a single nephron. Students often have difficulty conceptualizing the tubulointerstitum of the kidney and the location of the peritubular capillaries that return substances that have been reabsorbed from the tubules into the extracellular fluid in the vascular compartment.

Figure 31-7 illustrates the mechanisms of reabsorption and secretion in urine formation.

—Glossary terms

basement membrane

blood urea nitrogen (BUN)

collecting tubules

cortex

creatinine clearance

cystoscopy

distal tubule

diuretics (aldosterone antagonists, loop, osmotic, thiazide)

epithelium

filtration

glomerulus

hilus

juxtaglomerular complex

loop of Henle

medulla

mesangium

nephron

podocytes

renal threshold

secretion

specific gravity

transport maximum

—Other teaching strategies

A. Obtain a beef or pork kidney from the meat department and section it so that students can observe kidney structures.

B. Obtain a urinometer and have students perform specific gravity on a urine specimen and compare it to the specific gravity of water.

Chapter 32

Alterations in Renal Function

Chapter 32 describes alterations in kidney structure and function. The chapter is divided into 6 parts: congenital disorders of the kidney, obstructive disorders, urinary tract infections, disorders of glomerular function, tubulointerstitial disorders, and neoplasm. The discussion of urinary tract infections includes both lower and upper urinary tract infections; it includes recent information related to host-agent interactions. Also included in the section on urinary tract infections is a discussion of normal changes in urinary tract function that occur during pregnancy and factors that predispose the pregnant woman to the development of urinary tract infections. The chapter also includes a discussion of proposed immune mechanisms in the development of glomerular disease and drug-related renal disease.

Teaching strategies

—Overhead transparencies

Figure 32-1 illustrates the location and causes of urinary tract obstructions.

—Glossary terms

agenesis

albuminuria

anuria

bacteriuria

cystitis

extracorporeal shock wave lithotripsy

glomerulosclosis

glomerulonephritis

horse shoe kidney

hydronephrosis

hypoalbuminemia

hypogenesis

lipiduria

membranous

nephroblastoma

nephrotic syndrome

nephritic syndromes

oliguria

polycystic kidney disease

proliferative

pyelonephritis

reflux

renal calculi

renal colic

sclerotic

tubulointerstitial

ureterovesical reflux

washout phenomenon

Wilms' tumor

Chapter 33

Renal Failure

Chapter 33 focuses on causes and manifestations of acute and chronic renal failure. The chapter includes discussions of: altered sexual functioning in persons with end-stage renal disease, the effect of renal failure on elimination of drugs, dialysis and renal transplantation as treatment methods for persons with end-stage renal disease, dietary management for persons with renal insufficiency, maintenance hemodialysis, maintenance continuous ambulatory dialysis, and initial post-transplantation.

Teaching Strategies

—Glossary terms

azotemia

end-stage renal
  disease

hemodialysis

intrarenal

osteodystrophy

peritoneal dialysis

postrenal

prerenal

renal impairment

renal insufficiency

uremia

—Other teaching strategies

Obtain a membrane coil from a hemodialysis dialysis machine for students to examine.

Examination questions

1. The use of milliequivalents when discussing fluid and electrolytes allows for rapid comparison of:

    a. molecular weights
    • b. ions or electrical charges
    c. osmotic forces

2. Serum osmolality is controlled by the:

    • a. plasma proteins
    b. red blood cells
    c. serum sodium concentration
    d. white blood cells

3. The Normal (average) urine output in the adult is:

    a. 20 cc/hr
    • b. 60 cc/hr
    c. 80 cc/hr
    d. 100 cc/hr

4. The most reliable method for assessing body water is:

    • a. change in body weight
    b. intake and output
    c. tissue turgor
    d. serum sodium levels

5. Insensible water losses are those that occur as the result of water that is lost in:

    a. urine and bowel movements
    • b. breathing and sweating
    c. vomitus and bowel movements
    d. urine

6. Compared to the adult, infants tolerate fluid deprivation poorly because of their:

    a. higher metabolic rate and smaller surface area
    b. immature kidney structures and smaller extracellular fluid volume
    • c. higher metabolic rate, larger surface area, and lesser ability to concentrate their urine
    d. greater percentage of extracellular fluid and lesser metabolic rate

7. Drugs that decrease antidiuretic hormone levels include:

    • a. ethanol and morphine antagonists
    b. thiazide diuretics and anesthetic agents
    c. tricylic antidepressants and meperidine
    d. chlorpropamide and phenobarbital

8. In diabetes inspidius, there is

    • a. increased elimination of a dilute urine
    b. decreased urination with concentrated urine
    c. an increase in serum osmolality resulting from an elevated blood sugar
    d. increased serum sodium resulting from increased aldosterone levels

9. The major physiologic stimulus for thirst is:

    a. polyurina
    b. hyponatremia
    • c. increased serum osmolality
    d. hypoglycemia

10. Third-space fluid losses are those that result from:

    a. excessive urine output
    b. excessive respiratory losses
    c. excessive sweating
 • d. sequesting of fluid in an area of the body that does not participate in extracellular fluid exchange

11. Which of the following signs would indicate a fluid deficit:

    a. acute weight loss and increase in blood pressure
 • b. decreased urine output, acute loss of body weight, weakness, and dry skin and mucus membranes
    c. physical weakness, weight gain, dry skin, and decreased urine output
    d. dry fissured tongue, rapid respirations, weight gain, and confusion or delirium

12. The neurologic manifestations of hyponatremia are related to:

 • a. swelling of neurons
    b. removal of water from neurons

13. Serum sodium level should always be evaluated in relation to:

    a. serum potassium levels
    b. acid-base balance
 • c. serum osmolality and body water levels
    d. serum chloride levels

14. Hypoaldosteronism is characterized by:

    a. increased sodium losses
    b. increased sodium losses and retention of potassium
    c. increased potassium losses
 • d. sodium retention and increased potassium losses

15. A major function of potassium is:

    a. maintenance of extracellular osmolality
 • b. regulation of the resting membrane potential of neuromuscular and other excitable tissue
    c. participation in the blood clotting process
    d. to serve as a buffer for acid-base balance

16. Normally the greatest losses of potassium occurs through the:

    a. skin
    b. bowels
 • c. kidneys
    d. lungs

17. The signs and symptoms of hypokalemia include:

 • a. polyuria and postural hypotension
    b. decreased urine output with high specific gravity and respiratory acidosis
    c. hypertension and metabolic acidosis
    d. respiratory alkalosis and paresthesias

18. Which one of the following observations is essential before a potassium-containing intravenous infusion is started on a severely traumatized patient:

    a. heart rate and blood pressure
 • b. urine output
    c. respiratory rate
    d. level of consciousness

19. The active form of calcium in terms of neuromuscular functioning is:

 • a. ionized calcium
    b. protein bound calcium
    c. calcium citrate

20. A major manifestation of hypocalcemia (Ca^{++}) is:

• a. increased neural excitability
   b. decreased neural excitability
   c. decreased blood clotting
   d. increased blood clotting

21. The signs and symptoms of magnesium deficit are similar to those associated with:

• a. hypercalcemia
   b. hypernatremia
   c. hyperkalemia
   d. hyperphosphatemia

22. Edema represents an increase in:

   a. intracellular fluid
• b. interstitial fluid
   c. intravascular fluid

23. The hydrostatic pressure in the vascular system results from:

• a. the effects of gravity
   b. the pumping action of the heart
   c. the skeletal muscle pumps
   d. the presence of nondiffusible plasma proteins

24. The mechanism whereby disorders of the lymphatic system contribute to edema formation is:

• a. failure to remove excess fluid and osmotically active substances from the extracellular spaces
   b. altered immune function resulting in increased capillary permeability
   c. a resultant obstruction of venous outflow
   d. a resultant increase in capillary pressure

25. The failure to pull fluids back into the capillary is a cause of edema in which one of the following conditions:

   a. increased capillary pressure due to congestive heart failure
   b. surgical removal of the lymphatic nodes and channels due to cancer of the breast
• c. impaired plasma protein synthesis due to liver failure
   d. increased capillary permeability due to an inflammatory response

26. Pitting edema occurs when:

• a. the amount of interstitial fluid exceeds the absorptive capacity of the tissue gel
   b. there is coagulation of serum proteins that are present in the interstitial spaces
   c. lymphatic flow from an area is interrupted
   d. the skin and tissue fibers have been stretched due to prolonged periods of edema

27. The main source of serum bicarbonate is:

   a. absorption of dietary bicarbonate
• b. carbon dioxide resulting from cellular metabolism
   c. medications containing sodium bicarbonate
   d. synthesis by the liver

28. Metabolic acidosis is defined as:

• a. a decrease in bicarbonate
   b. an increase in bicarbonate
   c. an increase in carbonic acid
   d. a decrease in carbonic acid

29. Which one of the following statements is true as it relates to acid-base balance:

- a. renal mechanisms for correcting an acid-base imbalance are less rapid than respiratory mechanisms but they continue to function until pH has been returned to a normal or near-normal range
  b. pH provides an accurate measure of serum bicarbonate and carbonic acid levels
  c. the acid-base buffer systems of the body consist of a weak acid and strong base
  d. the body uses respiratory compensatory mechanisms to prevent large changes in pH resulting from respiratory disease

30. Among the causes of metabolic acidosis are:

- a. uncontrolled diabetes mellitus and severe exercise
  b. hyperventilation and hypokalemia
  c. chronic lung disease and hypochloremia
  d. drug overdose and hypokalemia

31. Acidosis usually causes:

- a. a decrease in central nervous system activity
  b. an increase in central nervous system activity

32. The reason that neurologic manifestations do not occur until late in the course of metabolic alkalosis is:

  a. an increase in pH does not affect neural function
- b. the bicarbonate ion does not readily cross the blood-brain barrier
  c. changes in ventilation prevent large changes in pH
  d. chloride ions compensate for the increased bicarbonate levels

33. In a person with a serum bicarbonate level of 12 mEq/L and PCO_2 20 mm Hg (carbonic acid 0.6 mEq/L) you would expect the pH to be:

- a. 7.4
  b. less than 7.4
  c. greater than 7.4

34. The overall function of the kidneys is to:

  a. eliminate water
  b. eliminate electrolytes
- c. regulate the composition of the extracellular fluid
  d. eliminate metabolic acids and conserve bicarbonate

35. Which one of the following diagnostic measures is used to assess the ability of the kidneys to concentrate urine:

  a. urine albumin
  b. urine pH
- c. urine specific gravity
  d. urine output

36. The antidiuretic hormone acts at the level of which one of the following kidney structures to increase urine concentration:

  a. glomerulus
  b. proximal tubule
  c. loop of Henle
- d. collecting tubule

37. Which one of the following blood tests is used as a measure of glomerular filtration rate and renal function:

  a. blood urea nitrogen
- b. serum creatinine
  c. serum potassium
  d. serum ammonia

38. Aspirin is not recommended for pain relief in persons with gouty arthritis because it:

    a. causes uric acid to precipitate in the urine
    • b. decreases the secretion of uric acid into the renal tubules
    c. increases uric acid synthesis by the kidneys
    d. decreases the filtration of uric acid in the glomeruli

39. The part of the kidney that receives the least blood flow is the:

    a. cortex
    b. medulla
    • c. papillae

40. The endocrine functions of the kidney include:

    a. activation of aldosterone and vitamin D
    • b. activation of angiotensin I, vitamin D, and erythropoietin
    c. activation of angiotensin II, vitamin D, and erythropoietin
    d. synthesis of vitamin D and erythropoietin

41. Which type of diuretic does not cause increased potassium losses:

    a. thiazide diuretics
    b. loop diuretics
    • c. aldosterone antagonists
    d. inhibitors of urine acidification

42. The most common complication of urinary tract obstruction is:

    a. incontinence
    • b. infection
    c. hypertension
    d. stone formation

43. Kidney damage resulting from urinary tract obstruction is usually the result of:

    • a. back pressure and ischemia
    b. infection
    c. irritation from urine stasis
    d. hypertension

44. Etiologic factors in the development of urolithiasis include:

    a. low antidiuretic hormone levels
    b. osmotic diuresis
    • c. urinary stasis
    d. high levels of sodium in the urine

45. Which type of kidney stone occurs more commonly in persons with urinary tract infections:

    a. calcium phosphate stones
    b. calcium oxalate stones
    • c. magnesium ammonium phosphate stones
    d. uric acid stones

46. Which one of the following would be included as a treatment measure for all types of kidney stones:

    a. acidification of urine
    b. decrease dietary intake of calcium
    c. prevention or treatment of urinary tract infections
    • d. increased fluid intake

47. The most common cause of nosocomial urinary tract infections is:

    a. decreased fluid intake
    • b. catheterization
    c. infrequent toileting
    d. improper or inadequate cleansing of the perineal area

48. Physiologic changes during pregnancy that contribute to the development of urinary tract infections include:

   a. decreased fluid intake due to first trimester nausea and vomiting
   • b. dilation of the collecting system of the kidneys and decreased peristalsis of the ureters
   c. increased bladder distention due to decreased filling sensation
   d. the presence of increased metabolic wastes from the placentofetal circulation that are in the urine

49. Glomerulonephritis is thought to result from:

   a. direct infection of the kidney
   b. renal trauma
   • c. an immune response

50. The edema that develops in persons with glomerulonephritis reflects

   a. impaired lymphatic function
   b. a decrease in capillary filtration pressure
   • c. a loss of plasma proteins
   d. a decrease in vascular volume

51. Pyelonephritis is a kidney disorder that involves the:

   a. glomerulus
   b. tubular epithelium only
   • c. tubular structures and the interstitium of the kidney
   d. ureters

52. Proliferative glomerular disease involves:

   • a an increase in the cells in the glomeruli
   b. an increase in the noncellular components of the glomeruli

53. The nephrotic syndrome is characterized by:

   a. hypertension, proteinuria, and hematuria
   • b. proteinuria, lipiduria, hypoalbuminemia, hyperlipidemia, and generalized edema
   c. proteinuria, hypertension, and generalized edema
   d. proteinuria, hypoalbuminemia, and generalized edema

54. One of the early signs of polycystic kidney disease is:

   a. polyuria
   b. hypertension
   c. proteinuria
   • d. enlarged kidneys

55. Which one of the following age groups are most susceptible to renal damage due to drugs:

   a. small children
   b. young adults
   c. middle-aged adults
   • d. elderly adults

56. Acute tubular necrosis is characterized by:

   • a. destructive changes in the tubular epithelium
   b. intratubular obstructions
   c. post-tubular obstruction
   d. acute swelling of the glomeruli

57. Most cases of acute tubular necrosis are caused by:

   a. acute glomerulonephritis
   • b. ischemia or nephrotoxic agents
   c. pyelonephritis
   d. hypertension

58. From your knowledge of renal function, you should conclude that the kidney changes associated with renal failure are:

   a. unilateral
   • b. bilateral

59. Signs of chronic renal failure do not develop until the disease is far advanced. This can best be explained in terms of:

 • a. the great functional reserve of kidneys.
  b. clinical signs and symptoms occur only when the distal tubules are involved
  c. increased blood pressure is able to compensate for alterations in kidney function until such a time as most of the tubular cells have been destroyed

60. The decrease in pH that occurs in persons with renal failure can best be explained in terms of:

  a. increased production of organic acids
  b. decreased ability of the kidneys to eliminate bicarbonate
 • c. decreased ability of the kidney to excrete metabolic acids
  d. impaired cellular metabolism

61. Anemia frequently found in persons with chronic renal failure can best be explained in terms of:

 • a. failure of the kidneys to activate or produce erythropoietin
  b. excess loss of vitamin B-12 by the kidneys
  c. loss of hemoglobin in the urine
  d. insufficient retention of iron

62. Demineralization of bone is a frequent finding in renal insufficiency. This is believed to be caused by:

  a. metabolic acidosis which is frequently present in renal insufficiency
 • b. failure of the kidneys to eliminate phosphate and activate vitamin D
  c. atrophy of the parathyroid glands induced by the uremia
  d. elevated blood urea nitrogen levels which are present in renal failure

63. Serum potassium is usually elevated in renal failure. This could most likely be attributed to the fact that:

 • a. most potassium losses occur through the kidney
  b. potassium is the chief cation in the extracellular fluid
  c. potassium is absorbed in the kidney
  d. potassium is lost in the stool
  e. potassium is contained in blood urea nitrogen

64. The development of hypertension in a person with renal failure is largely related to:

  a. increased loss of albumin in the urine
 • b. increased intravascular fluid and the reninangiotension mechanism
  c. increased levels of ADH
  d. elevated blood urea nitrogen levels which are present in renal failure

65. The nocturia that often presents as an early symptom of renal failure can best be explained in terms of:

  a. loss of bladder tone
  b. decreased ability to excrete urine
 • c. loss of ability to concentrate urine
  d. increased filtering of water in the glomerulus

Alterations in Genitourinary Function

Unit 7 focuses on alterations in genitourinary function. The unit is divided into six chapter: Chapter 34, Alterations in Urine Elimination; Chapter 35, Structure and Function of the Male Genitourinary System; Chapter 36, alterations in Male Genitourinary Function; Chapter 37, Structure and Function of the Female Reproductive System; Chapter 38, Alterations in Structure and Function of the Female Reproductive System; and Chapter 39, Sexually Transmitted Diseases. Aging changes in male reproductive function are discussed in Chapter 35 and menopause in Chapter 37. Infertility is discussed in Chapter 38.

Chapter 34

Alterations in Urine Elimination

Although the kidneys control the formation of urine, it is the bladder that stores urine and regulates its elimination. Chapter 33 focuses on alterations in urine elimination. The chapter is organized into 3 sections: (1) control of urine elimination, (2) alterations in bladder function, and (3) cancer of the bladder. The chapter includes a discussion of urinary retention and urinary incontinence. The mechanisms of voiding in neurogenic bladder associated with spinal cord injury are introduced in this chapter and discussed further in Chapter 49.

Teaching strategies

—Glossary terms

autonomic hyperreflexia

catheterization

Crede's method

cystometerography

detrusor muscle

detrusor muscle areflexia

detrusor-sphincter dyssynergy

electromyography

frequency

hesitancy

incontinence (environmental or spurious, overflow, psychological, reflex, urge, stress)

residual urine

micturition center

muscarinic receptors

neurogenic bladder

nicotinic receptors

pelvic floor muscles

pelvic nerve

pudendal nerve

rugae

trigone

urethra

urethrovesicle angle

urination

urodynamic studies

uroflometry

vesicle

voiding

Chapter 35

Structure and Function of the Male Genitourinary System

Chapter 35 focuses on the structure and function of the male genitourinary system. The chapter is organized into 3 sections: (1) male genitourinary structures, (2) reproductive function, and (3) neural control of sexual function. The chapter ends with a discussion of changes in the male genitourinary system that occur with aging. The autonomic nervous system control of sexual function in the male is discussed further in Chapter 48.

Teaching strategies

—Overhead transparencies

Figure 35-2 illustrates the parts of the testis and epididymis.

Figure 35-3 shows the excretory ducts of the male reproductive system and the path that sperm follow as they leave the testes and travel to the urethra.

—Glossary terms

adenohyphysis	glans
cells of Leydig	gonads
cremaster muscle	gonatotropins
cryptorchidism	prepuce
ejaculation	semen
emission	sertoli cells
epididymis	spermatocytes
erection	spermatogenesis
foreskin	spermatogonia
genitourinary system	testes

Chapter 36

Alterations in Male Genitourinary Function

Chapter 36 focuses on alterations in male genitourinary function. The content in this chapter is arranged according to structure: (1) disorders of the penis, (2) disorders of the scrotum and testes, and (3) disorders of the prostate. The chapter includes a discussion of cancer of the penis, scrotum, testes, and prostate.

Teaching strategies

—Overhead transparencies

Figure 36-4 depicts a hydrocele and **Figure 36-5** testicular torsion.

—Glossary terms

choriocarcinoma	hydrocele
epididymitis	hyperplasia
epispadias	hypospadias
germ cell tumors	leukoplakia
hematocele	orchitis

Peyronie's disease	spermatocele
phimosis	teratoma
priapism	testicular torsion
prostatitis	varicocele
prostatodynia	

—Other teaching strategies

State the methods used in diagnosis and treatment of prostatic cancer.

Chapter 37

Structure and Function of the Female Reproductive System

Chapter 37 focuses on structure and function of the female reproductive system. The chapter is organized into three sections: (1) female reproductive structures, (2) the menstrual cycle, and (3) the breast. The chapter includes a discussion of the menopause.

Teaching strategies

—Overhead transparencies

Figure 37-1 shows the female reproductive system.

Figure 37-2 illustrates the external genitalia.

Figure 37-3 is a schematic diagram of the female organs and the pathway for the oocyte as it moves from the ovary into the fallopian tube.

Figure 37-8 shows the glandular tissue and ducts of the breast.

—Glossary terms

amenorrhea	fundus
androgens	genitalia
Bartholin's glands	introitus
cervix	labia
clitoris	mittelschmerz
corpus luteum	myometrium
dysmenorrhea	oogenesis
endometrium	perimetrium
estrogens	progesterone
ferning	prolactin
fimbriae	spinnbarkiet
follicles	vestibule
fornices	

Chapter 38

Alterations in Structure and Function of the Female Reproductive System

Chapter 38 focuses on alterations in structure and function of the female reproductive system. The chapter includes discussions of disorders of the female external genitalia, vagina, cervix, uterus, fallopian tubes and ovaries, and pelvic support and uterine position; menstrual disorders, and disorders of the breast. The chapter ends with a discussion of infertility that includes both male and female factors.

Teaching strategies

—Overhead transparency

Figure 38-5 illustrates the muscles of the pelvic floor.

—Glossary terms

adenomyosis

amenorrhea

anovulatory

cervical intraepithelial neoplasia (CIN)

cystocele

dysmenorrhea

endometriosis

endometritis

enterocele

ervicitis

fibroadenoma

fibrocystic disease

fibroid

folliculitis

galatorrhea

gamete intra-fallopian transfer

hypomenorrhea

hysterectomy

invitro fertilization

leiomyoma

mastitis

menometorrhagia

nabothian cyst

oligomenorrhea

Paget's disease

pelvic inflammatory disease (PID)

polycystic ovarian syndrome

rectocele

transformation zone

uterine prolapse

vaginitis

vulvitis

Chapter 39

Sexually Transmitted Diseases

Chapter 39 focuses on sexually transmitted diseases. The chapter is organized into 3 parts: (1) infections of the external genitalia, (2) vaginal infections, and (3) vaginal/urogenital/systemic infections.

Teaching strategies
—Glossary terms

candidiasis

chancroid

chlamydial infection

cryotherapy

granuloma inguinale

latency

neurotropic

spirocete

trichomonas vaginalis

varicella-zoster virus

Examination questions

1. The reflex control of bladder emptying occurs at the level of the:

   a. cerebral cortex
   b. medulla
   c. thoracolumbar spinal cord
   ● d. sacral spinal cord

2. Sympathetic stimulation of the bladder causes:

   ● a. relaxation of the detrusor muscle and contraction of the internal sphincter
   b. contraction of the detrusor muscle and relaxation of the internal sphincter
   c. contraction of the detrusor muscle and contraction of the internal sphincter
   d. relaxation of the detrusor muscle and relaxation of the internal sphincter

3. Which one of the following drug groups act to decrease external sphincter tone:

   a. cholinergic drugs
   b. anticholinergic drugs
   c. adrenergic blocking drugs
   ● d. skeletal muscle relaxants

4. The early stages of obstruction to urine outflow from the bladder is manifested by:

   ● a. frequency and urgency
   b. temporary interruption in voiding before complete emptying can be accomplished
   c. secondary infection due to urine stasis
   d. complete retention of urine

5. Following a stroke that affects the cortex or pyramidal tract:

   a. storage reflexes are provoked during filling and uninhibited bladder contractions occur at lower volumes and at increased external sphincter tone
   ● b. the ability to perceive bladder filling is lost and voiding occurs suddenly and without warning
   c. the bladder fills but does not contract
   d. there is overfilling of the bladder with a lack of appreciation of bladder events

6. No more than 1000 ml of urine should be removed during acute overdistention of the bladder because of the danger of:

   a. damage to the bladder wall
   ● b. shock due to the sudden release of pressure on pelvic blood vessels
   c. urinary tract infection
   d. reflux of urine into the ureters and bladder

7. Bladder retraining that uses the Crede method focuses on:

   a. trigger point methods that stimulate the afferent loop of the voiding reflex
   b. frequent toileting to prevent overdistention of the bladder
   ● c. the use of suprapubic pressure to increase intravesicular pressure and promote bladder emptying
   d. the use of biofeedback methods to train a person to raise intravesicular pressure

8. Stress incontinence is characterized by:

   a. involuntary loss of urine due to abnormal activity of the micturition centers in the sacral cord
   ● b. involuntary loss of urine associated with activities such coughing or squatting
   c. awareness of the need to urinate but failure to respond appropriately
   d. involuntary loss of urine when intravesicular pressure exceeds urethral pressure in the absence of detrusor activity

9. Conditions that are associated with overflow incontinence include:

   a. upper motor neuron lesions and musculoskeletal disorders
   ● b. prostatic obstruction and fecal impaction
   c. treatment with drugs such as hynotics and tranquilizers
   d. childbirth and surgical procedures that weaken the muscles of the pelvic floor

10. The most common sign of bladder cancer is:

   a. incontinence
   b. urine retention
   ● c. hematuria
   d. dysuria

11. Testosterone is produced by the:

   a. sertoli cells
   b. seminal vesicle
   ● c. cells of Leydig
   d. ductus deferens

12. The production of testosterone is regulated by:

   ● a. LH
   b. FSH

13. Gonadotrophin-stimulated production of testosterone normally begins at about age:

   a. 2 to 4 years
   b. 4 to 6 years
   ● c. 10 to 12 years
   d. 18 to 21 years

14. The function of the scrotum is to:

   a. produce sperm
   b. produce testosterone
   ● c. enclose and regulate the temperature of the testes
   d. transport sperm

15. The small unspecialized germinal cells that characterize the firststage of spermatogenesis are called:

   a. primary spermatocytes
   ● b. spermatogonia
   c. spermatids
   d. spermatozoon

16. Mature sperm are normally stored in the:

   a. epididymis
   ● b. vas deferens
   c. seminal vesicle
   d. prostatic urethra

17. Afferent impulses from the sensory receptors in the glans penis enter the central nervous system at the level of the:

   ● a. sacral cord
   b. lumbar cord
   c. thoracic cord
   d. cervical cord

18. In males with hypospadias, the termination of the urethra is on the:

   ● a. ventral surface of the penis
   b. dorsal surface of the penis
   c. lateral surface of the penis

19. Priapism is characterized by:

    a. a hard fibrous plaque in the shaft of the penis
  • b. prolonged painful erection
    c. failure of the testes to descend into the scrotum
    d. tightening of the penile foreskin

20. Which one of the following hormones may be used to stimulate descent of the testes in children with cryptorchidism:

    a. testosterone
    b. follicle-stimulating hormone
    c. luteinizing hormone
  • d. Gonadotrophin Releasing Hormone (GRH)

21. In a hydrocele, excess fluid is present in the:

    a. seminal vesicles
    b. epididymis
  • c. tunica vaginalis
    d. vas deferens

22. The immediate complications of testicular torsion are related to:

    a. impaired sexual function
    b. impaired testosterone production
    c. infertility
  • d. impaired blood flow

23. The manifestations of epididymitis include:

  • a. unilateral pain and swelling of the testes
    b. bilateral testicular pain and erythema of the overlying scrotum
    c. abnormal feeling of heaviness in the left scrotum
    d. accumulation of blood in the scrotum

24. The American Cancer Society recommends that testicular self exam should be done:

    a. every week
  • b. once a month
    c. twice a year
    d. whenever there is scrotal or testicular discomfort

25. Which one of the following germ cell tumors is thought to be derived from the seminiferous epithelium in the testes:

    a. choriocarcinoma
  • b. seminoma
    c. teratoma
    d. embryonal carcinoma

26. A common symptoms of benign prostatic hyperplasia is:

  • a. decreased force and caliber of the urinary stream
    b. suprapubic pain
    c. burning on urination
    d. painful erection

27. The major significance of benign prostatic hypertrophy is its ability to:

    a. progress to prostatic cancer
    b. impair sexual function
  • c. cause urinary obstruction
    d. predispose to prostatitis

28. The incidence of prostatic cancer is greatest in men:

    a. between the ages of 20 and 30 years
    b. between the ages of 40 and 60 years
  • c. over age 65
    d. over age 75

29. The location of the skenes glands is:

    a. between the hymenal opening and posterior labia minora
    ● b. at the urethra opening
    c. at the anterior labia minora
    d. in the vagina between the hymenal opening and the cervix

30. The cul-de-sac is formed by which one of the following uterine layers:

    ● a. perimetrium
    b. myometrium
    c. endometrium

31. Dysmenorrhea originates in the:

    a. perimetrium
    ● b. myometrium
    c. endometrium

32. Oogenesis or generation of the primordial ova by mitotic division occurs during:

    ● a. fetal life
    b. early childhood
    c. menarche
    d. each monthly cycle

33. The source of estrogens is:

    ● a. ovaries and adipose tissue
    b. ovaries and the anterior pituitary gland
    c. the ovaries only

34. The secretion of FSH and LH is under the direct control of:

    a. estrogen
    b. thyroxin
    c. oxytocin
    ● d. gonadotrophin-releasing factor

35. Which type of estrogen is the most abundantly secreted product of the ovary and has the greatest biological activity:

    ● a. estradiol
    b. estrone
    c. estriol

36. Progesterone is produced by the:

    a. granulosa cells of the ovary
    ● b. corpus luteum of the ovary
    c. anterior pituitary gland
    d. adrenal gland

37. The actions of progesterone include:

    a. promotion of ovarian follicle growth
    ● b. promotion of the cyclic glandular development of the endometrium
    c. proliferation and cornification of vaginal mucosa
    d. contribute to the growth of axillary and pubic hair

38. The absence of ferning of the cervical mucus suggests:

    a. insufficient progesterone secretion
    ● b. inadequate estrogen stimulation of the endocervical glands
    c. anovulatory cycles

39. Milk is produced by the:

    a. ductile tissue of the breast
    ● b. alveolar tissue of the breast

40. The hormone responsible for ejection of milk into the ductal system of the breast is:

    a. estrogen
    b. progesterone
    c. prolactin
    ● d. oxytocin

41. In its initial stages, cancer of the vulva often appears as:

    ● a. a thickening of the vulvar skin
    b. an ulcerated nodular lesion
    c. a flat ulcerated lesion with persistent drainage
    d. a painful nodular lesion

42. The transformation zone in the cervix can be described as:

   • a. the area of metaplasia where columnar cells of endocervix are transformed to squamous epithelium
   b. normal junction between the columnar cells of the exocervix and the squamous cells of the vagina
   c. an area of cancer insitu of the cervix
   d. the area that joins the vagina and the cervix

43. The pap smear that examines cells from the surface of the cervix and endocervix is used to detect:

   a. normal and cancerous cells
   b. normal and precancerous cells
   • c. both precancerous and cancerous cells

44. Endometriosis can be described as a condition in which:

   a. there is inflammation of the endometrium
   • b. functional endometrial tissue is found in ectopic sites outside the uterus
   c. endometrial glands and stroma are found within the myometrium

45. A contributing factor in the development of endometrial cancer is thought to be:

   a. sexually transmitted viruses
   • b. abnormal hormone levels
   c. early age of first intercourse and multiple sexual partners
   d. frequent vaginal infections

46. The greatest danger associated with tubal pregnancy is:

   a. abortion
   b. fetal abnormalities
   • c. tubal rupture

47. A cystocele involves:

   • a. herniation of the bladder into the vagina
   b. herniation of the rectum into the bladder
   c. bulging of the uterus into the vagina
   d. anterior flexion of the uterus so that rests on the bladder

48. Menometrorrhagia describes a condition in which there is:

   a. bleeding between menstrual periods
   b. heavy bleeding during the menstrual period
   • c. heavy bleeding both during and between menstrual periods
   d. irregular menstrual periods

49. Most breast cancers are discovered through use of:

   a. physician exams
   b. mammography
   • c. breast self-exam
   d. chest x-rays

50. A surge in which one of the gonadotrophic hormones is necessary for ovulation to occur:

   a. FSH
   • b. LH
   c. prolactin

51. In an ovulatory cycle, basal body temperature is increased:

   a. during the follicular phase just prior to ovulation
   • b. during the luteal phase that follows ovulation
   c. during menstruation
   d. just prior to menstruation

52. Which one of the following sexually transmitted diseases has systemic as well as genitourinary manifestations:

    a. condylomata accuminata
    b. recurrent genital herpes
    c. trichomonas
 • d. gonorrhea

53. A major concern related to condyloma accuminata (genital warts) is their:

    a. ability to cause disfigurement
 • b. association with premalignant and malignant genital lesions
    c. tendency for the lesions to become infected
    d. association with infertility

54. Recurrent genital herpes infections result from:

    a. an immune response arising from repeated exposure to the virus
 • b. activation of the virus which is maintained in a latency state in neurons of the sacral dorsal root ganglia
    c. activation of the virus which is maintained in a latency state in the genital tissues
    d. reinfection with herpes simplex type I virus

55. Candidiasis is caused by what type of microorganism?

    a. a virus
 • b. a yeast
    c. a bacteria
    d. a protozoan

56. The reason that antibiotic therapy predisposes to vulvovaginal candiasis is that it:

    a. produces a decrease in immune function
 • b. suppresses the normal protective flora
    c. decreases the pH of vaginal secretions
    d. increases vaginal glycogen stores

57. Which one of the following types of vaginal discharge is characteristic of a trichomonas infection:

    a. thin and watery
 • b. copious frothy green or yellow and foul smelling
    c. homogenous fishy smelling with a pH above 4.5
    d. mucopurulent

58. A serious complication of chlamydial infections in women is:

    a. cervicitis and increased risk of cervical cancer
 • b. pelvic inflammatory disease and infertility or ectopic pregnancy
    c. urinary frequency and dysuria
    d. endometriosis

Alterations in Metabolism, Endocrine Function, and Nutrition

Unit 8 focuses on alterations in gastrointestinal function, nutritional status, and endocrine control of growth and metabolism. The unit includes Chapters 39, 40, and 41 which focus on the gastrointestinal tract and alterations in digestive function. Chapter 42 presents a discussion of energy metabolism, nutritional status, obesity, and malnutrition. The mechanisms of endocrine control of body function are discussed in Chapter 43 and alterations in endocrine control of growth and metabolism in Chapter 44. Because of its importance as a major health problem that affects all age groups, an entire chapter (Chapter 45) has been devoted to diabetes mellitus.

Chapter 40

Control of Gastrointestinal Function

The digestive system is truly an amazing structure. In this system, enzymes and hormones are produced, vitamins are synthesized and stored, and food is dismantled and then reassembled. Structurally, the gastrointestinal system is a long, hollow tube with its lumen inside the body and its wall acting as an interface between the internal and external environments. Although not a part of the gastrointestinal tract, the salivary glands, liver, and pancreas function as accessory organs for the digestive system.

Chapter 40 focuses on control of gastrointestinal function. The chapter is organized into 4 sections: (1) structure and organization of the gastrointestinal tract, (2) gastrointestinal motility, (3) secretory function, and (4) digestion and absorption. The function of the liver, gall bladder, and exocrine pancreas is integrated into Chapter 41.

Teaching strategies

—Overhead transparencies

Figure 40-1 depicts the digestive system.

Figure 40-5 shows the four main layers of the wall of the digestive tract.

Figure 40-7 shows the autonomic innervation of the gastrointestinal tract.

—Glossary terms

alimentary canal	digestive tract
bowel	enterocytes
chief cells	gastrin
cholecystokinin	gut
crypts of Leiberkuhn	haustrations
defecation	intraluminal

mass movements

mesentery

myenteric
  (Auerbach's plexus)

omentum

parietal cells

parietal peritoneum

pepsinogen

peristalsis

peritoneum

pylorus

secretin

segmentation waves

sphincter

steatorrhea

submucosal
  (Meissner's plexus)

villi

visceral peritoneum

—Other teaching strategies

Use a balloon to illustrate the enclosure of the bowel in the peritoneum (see **Figure 39-3**).

Chapter 41

Alterations in Gastrointestinal Function

Normal gastrointestinal function requires an intact mucosal surface, motility that moves the contents forward, and digestion of foods and their absorption through the wall of the digestive tract. Chapter 40 focuses on alterations in gastrointestinal function. The chapter is organized into four sections: (1) manifestations of gastrointestinal disorders, (2) alterations in the integrity of the gastrointestinal tract, (3) alterations in motility, and (4) malabsorption. The section on manifestations of gastrointestinal disorders provides a discussion of anorexia, nausea, vomiting, and gastrointestinal bleeding which are frequent manifestations of gastrointestinal pathology.

Teaching strategies

—Glossary terms

achalasia

anorexia

cathartic

colonoscopy

constipation

Crohn's disease

Curling's ulcer

Cushing's ulcer

diarrhea (large and
  small volume)

dissacharides

diverticulosis

dumping syndrome

dysphagia

esophagitis

fecal impaction

gastritis

glossitis

H_2-receptor
  antagonists

heartburn

hematemesis

hiatal hernia

inflammatory bowel
  disease

intussusception

luminal

malabsorption

melena

monosaccarides

nausea

paralytic ileus

peptic ulcer

peritonitis

proctosigmoidoscopy

reflux

strangulated hernia

ulcerative colitis

vomiting

Zollinger-Ellison
  syndrome

—Other teaching strategies

A. Have students evaluate the contents of over-the-counter antacids in terms of contraindications and possible side effects.

Chapter 42

Alterations in Function of the Hepatobiliary System and Exocrine Pancreas

The liver, gall bladder, and pancreas are classified as accessory organs of the digestive system. In addition to producing digestive secretions, both the liver and pancreas have other important functions. The endocrine pancreas assists in storage and release of energy substrates through the production and release of insulin and glucagon. The liver synthesizes glucose, plasma proteins, and clotting factors and is responsible for the degradation and elimination of drugs and hormones.

Chapter 41 focuses on alterations in function of the hepatobiliary and exocrine pancreas. The chapter is organized into four sections: hepatobiliary function, alterations in liver function, alterations in gallbladder function, and alterations in function of the exocrine pancreas. Alterations in the endocrine pancreas function—diabetes mellitus—is discussed in Chapter 45.

Teaching strategies

—Overhead transparencies

Figure 42-2 depicts portal circulation.

Figure 42-2 illustrates the structures of a liver lobule.

—Glossary terms

ampulla of Vater	hepatic encephalopathy
ascites	hepatitis
asterixis	hepatobiliary
autodigestion	hepatomegaly
bile acids	icterus
bilirubin	jaundice
cholecystitis	kernicterus
cholecystography	portal hypertension
choleliathiasis	pseudocyst
cholescintigraphy	purpura
cirrhosis	splenogaly
conjugated	telangiectasia
esophageal varices	urobilogen
fetor hepaticus	

Chapter 43

Alterations in Nutritional Status

Nutritional status describes the condition of the body as it relates to the availability and utilization of nutrients. Nutrients provide the energy and materials necessary for performing the activities of daily living; for maintaining healthy skin, muscles, and other body tissues; for replacing and healing tissues; and for the effective functioning of all body systems including the immune and respiratory systems. Chapter 42 focuses on alterations in nutritional status. The chapter is organized into 3 sections: (1) nutritional status, (2) overnutrition and obesity, and undernutrition.

Teaching strategies

—Overhead transparency

Figure 43-2 shows the regulation of blood glucose by the liver. Recent evidence suggests that the distribution of body fat may be a more important factor for morbidity and mortality than the mere presence of overweight status.

—Glossary terms

adipose tissue

amino acid

amino group

anabolism

android

anthropometric

basal energy equivalent (BEE)

basal metabolic rate (BMR)

body mass index (BMI)

bulimarexia

bulimia

cachexia

calorie

carbohydrate

catabolism

densitometry

dietary fiber

emetic

energy

fatty acid

gluconeogenesis

glucose

glycerol

glycogenolysis

gynoid

ketones

kwashikor

marasmus

metabolism

metabolites

minerals

nutrient

obesity (upper body and lower body obesity)

purging behaviors

recommended daily allowances (RDA)

thermogenesis

triglyceride

vitamins

—Other teaching strategies

Have students describe their weight status using the Metropolitan Height and Weight Tables, BMI, and weight-ratio; have them analyze their energy expenditures using Table 42-2; and caloric requirements using Table 42-4.

Chapter 44

Mechanisms of Endocrine Control

Chapter 44 focuses on the mechanisms of endocrine control and is intended as an introduction to Chapters 44 and 45. The chapter is organized into two parts: the first part discusses the endocrine system and hormones, while the second part covers general aspects of endocrine function.

Teaching Strategies

—Overhead Transparency

Figure 44-4 depicts hypothalamic-pituitary-target cell feedback mechanisms.

—Glossary Terms

amine

bioassay

glycoprotein

hormone

hypophysis

hypothalamus

polypetide

prohormone

radioimmunoassay

receptor affinity and binding

second messenger

steroid

target cell

Chapter 45

Alterations in Endocrine Control of Growth and Metabolism

Chapter 45 focuses on endocrine control of growth and metabolism. The chapter is organized into 3 sections: (1) growth and growth hormone disorders, (2) thyroid disorders, and (3) disorders of adrenal cortical function. Other material, pertinent to the content of this chapter, can be found in the following chapters: Chapter 45 focuses on insulin and diabetes mellitus, Chapter 27 on antidiuretic hormone, and Chapter 56 on alterations in calcium metabolism and its effect on skeletal function. Testosterone and its

function in the male are discussed in Chapter 34 and estrogen and progesterone on the female in Chapter 36.

Teaching Strategies

—Overhead Transparency

Figure 45-2 can be used to illustrate the thyroid gland and its follicular structure.

—Glossary Terms

acromegaly

Addison's disease

adrenal hyperplasia

adrenogenital syndrome

biosynthesis

catch-up growth

constitutional short and tall stature

cortisol

cretinism

Cushing's syndrome

diiodotyrosine

euthyroid

exophthalmos

glucocorticoid hormones

goiter

Graves' disease

hormone (somatotropin)

hyperpigmentation

mineralocorticoids

monoiodotyrosine

mucopolysaccharide

myxedema

panhypopituitarism

sella turcica

somatomedins

somatostatin

stature (short and tall)

striae thyroid follicle

thyrotoxicosis

thyroxine

triiodothyronine

Chapter 46

Diabetes Mellitus

Because diabetes mellitus is a common health problem, an entire chapter has been devoted to the disorder. Chapter 45 focuses on the role of insulin in glucose, protein, and fat metabolism and diabetes mellitus. The chapter is organized in 4 parts: (1) hormonal control of blood sugar, (2) classification and etiology of diabetes mellitus, (3) manifestations of diabetes mellitus, and (4) diagnosis and management of diabetes mellitus.

Teaching Strategies

—Glossary Terms

exchange diet

gestational diabetes

glucose tolerance

glycosuria

glycosylated hemoglobin

hyperglycemia

hyperosmolar

hypoglycemia

insulin-dependent diabetes (IDDM)

ketoacidosis

ketosis

labile diabetes

nephropathy

neuropathy

noninsulin-dependent diabetes (NIDDM)

photocoagulation

polydipsia

polyol

polyphagia

polyuria

retinopathy (proliferative, background)

secondary diabetes

Somogyi phenomenon

vulvovaginitis

—Other Teaching Strategies

A. Have students do capillary blood glucose measurement. You may want to demonstrate the effect of improper skin preparation by having students apply a drop of rubbing alcohol to the reagent strip rather than blood and observe the 'glucose' reading. Discuss universal precautions in terms of lancet use and disposal for blood glucose screening projects.

B. Assign students to use the exchange system for diet management to select food for their meals for a day (you may want to include lunch at a fast food establishment or dinner at a restaurant).

C. Have students explain the difference in control of blood sugar in a person without diabetes and in a person with insulin-dependent diabetes mellitus who is in good control (normal blood sugar at the onset of exercise) and in poor control (presence of elevated blood sugar and ketoacidosis at the onset of exercise).

D. Have students discuss instructions for a person with insulin-dependent diabetes regarding insulin administration during gastrointestinal flu that entails nausea and vomiting.

E. Have students investigate the cost of glucose monitoring and insulin replacement therapy for a person with diabetes.

Examination Questions

1. The digestion and absorption of nutrients from the GI tract occurs mainly in the:

   a. stomach
   b. duodenum
   • c. jejunum and ileum
   d. colon

2. Which layer of the gastrointestinal tract wall heals by regeneration and without scar tissue replacement:

   • a. mucosal layer
   b. submucosal layer
   c. circular muscle layer
   d. longitudinal muscle layer

3. Normal peristalsis:

   a. consists of continuous tonic movements
   • b. moves in the direction from the mouth toward the anus
   c. is under the direct control of the central nervous system
   d. only occurs in the colon

4. Sympathetic innervation of the gastrointestinal tract:

   a. is distributed by way of the vagus nerve
   • b. inhibits gastrointestinal motility and enhances sphincter tone
   c. increases gastrointestinal secretions and motility
   d. is limited to the stomach and duodenum

5. Which one of the following hormones is involved in gastric acid secretion

   a. pepsinogen
   b. cholecystokinin
   c. secretin
   • d. gastrin

6. Brush border enzymes such as sucrase are produced by the:

   a. salivary glands
   b. gastric mucosal cells
   • c. enterocytes of the small intestine
   d. exocrine cells in the pancreas

7. A major symptom of lactase deficiency is:

   a. steatorrhea
   • b. flatulence and diarrhea
   c. constipation and bloating
   d. weight loss

8. Vomiting consists of the following sequence of events:

   a. forceful contraction of the diaphragm and abdominal muscles, closure of the airways, relaxation of the esophageal sphincter, and deep inspiration

   • b. deep inspiration, closure of the airways, forceful contraction of the diaphragm and abdominal muscles, and relaxation of the esophageal sphincter

   c. closure of the airways, forceful contraction of the diaphragm and abdominal muscles, deep inspiration, and relaxation of the esophageal sphincter

   d. relaxation of the esophageal sphincter, forceful contraction of the diaphragm and abdominal muscles, deep inspiration, and closure of the airways

9. The term melena refers to:

   a. blood in the vomitus
   b. gaseous distention of the bowel
   • c. blood in the stool
   d. loss of appetite

10. A common manifestation of a hiatal hernia is:

   • a. heartburn
   b. diarrhea
   c. belching
   d. difficulty swallowing

11. Etiologic factors in acute gastritis include:

   a. immune mechanisms
   b. excessive production of hydrochloric acid
   c. lack of the intrinsic factor
   • d. excessive alcohol consumption and other local irritants

12. Factors which contribute to the development of a peptic ulcer include:

   • a. disruption of the gastric mucosal barrier
   b. increased activity of Brunner's glands
   c. decreased gastric acid/pepsin production
   d. decreased movement of intestinal bile into the stomach

13. The therapeutic effect of histamine-2 receptor antagonists on peptic ulcer is related to the drugs ability to:

   a. bind to the gastric mucosa and serve as a protective barrier
   b. neutralize acid/pepsin secretions
   c. relieve anxiety and stress
   • d. block gastric acid secretion

14. The symptoms of the dumping syndrome (e.g., diaphoresis, tachycardia, and lightheadedness) that occur shortly after eating in some persons who have had a gastrojejunostomy are related to:

   a. increased small bowel activity
   • b. loss of vascular volume and hyperinsulinemia due to rapid movement of gastric contents into the small intestine
   c. increased acid/pepsin production
   d. disruption of the intestinal flora

15. Crohn's disease is characterized by:

   • a. sharply demarcated granulomatous skip lesions of the bowel
   b. ulcerative lesions of the mucosal layer of the colon
   c. increased risk of colon cancer
   d. lack of systemic involvement

16. Protective mechanisms that the body uses to control peritonitis following perforation of the bowel include:

    a. Increased blood flow to the bowel to allow for rapid absorption of contaminated materials from the perforated bowel

    • b. decreased peristalsis and formation of thick fibrous exudate to seal off the perforated bowel

    c. increased peristalsis and diarrhea to prevent stasis of bowel contents

    d. increased movement of fluid into the bowel in an effort to dilute toxins that are in the bowel contents

17. Which one of the following positions is used to prevent complications associated with abscess formation due to peritonitis:

    a. trendelenbury (head-down)

    b. supine with one pillow under the head

    • c. the head and knees elevated (semi-fowlers)

    d. lying on the left side (left lateral)

18. The reason that diverticulum occur primarily in the sigmoid colon is related to the fact that:

    • a. there is not a continuous longitudinal muscle layer in the sigmoid colon

    b. the diameter of the sigmoid colon is greater than other sections of the large bowel

    c. this section of the colon lacks the circular layer of muscle

    d. there are no regularly occurring peristaltic movements in the sigmoid colon

19. Small volume diarrhea is usually associated with:

    • a. inflammatory bowel disease

    b. acute infections that increase intestinal secretory activity

    c. ingestion of osmotic agents

    d. lactose intolerance

20. The major effects of small bowel obstruction are:

    • a. abdominal distention and loss of fluids and electrolytes

    b. diarrhea and vomiting

    c. constipation and fever

    d. abdominal pain and hypotension

21. The defecation urge:

    • a. occurs during mass movements in the colon

    b. occurs only in the morning and at night

    c. accompanies peristaltic movements of the small intestine

    d. requires conscious thought

22. Celiac disease involves the:

    • a. intestinal villi

    b. mucosal layer of the colon

    c. biliary ducts of the liver

    d. acinar cells of the pancreas

23. An early sign or symptom of cancer of the colon is:

    a. pain on defecation

    • b. change in bowel habits

    c. anorexia

    d. unexplained weight loss

24. Bilirubin is derived from:

    a. cholesterol metabolism

    b. bile salts

    • c. breakdown of senescent red blood cells

25. Early signs of jaundice are most easily observed in the:

    a. oral mucosa

    • b. sclera of the eye

    c. nail beds

    d. ear lobes

26. The alterations in liver function that occur with persons with cirrhosis are related to:

●   a. formation of bands of fibrous tissue that replace normal hepatic cells and distort the architecture of the liver

    b. excessive accumulation of fat within hepatocytes and biliary ducts

    c. localized injury to biliary ducts in the liver

    d. abnormal deposition of minerals within hepatic cells and biliary ducts

27. In cirrhosis, an increased blood ammonia level is related to impaired liver function as it relates to:

●   a. urea synthesis

    b. gluconeogenesis

    c. prothrombin production

    d. production of ketones

28. The encephalopathies or alterations in CNS function which appear late in the course of cirrhosis are associated with:

    a. impaired blood flow to the brain resulting from portal vein obstruction

●   b. failure of the liver to remove ammonia and metabolic wastes from the blood

    c. elevated levels of blood urea nitrogen

    d. elevated blood sugar levels

29. Factors which contribute to the development of cholelithiasis include:

●   a. stasis and altered composition of bile

    b. diabetes

    c. cirrhosis

    d. excess consumption of fatty foods

30. Surgical removal of the gallbladder would be expected to:

    a. decrease bile production by the liver

●   b. decrease the ability to store and concentrate bile

    c. produce a complete lack of bile to aid in digestion

    d. impair the passage of bile into the intestine

31. Acute pancreatitis results from:

    a. an infectious process

    b. ischemia

●   c. an autodigestive process

    d. an autoimmune response

32. Which one of the following serum enzymes becomes elevated during the the first 24 hours following the onset of acute pancreatitis:

●   a. amylase

    b. alkaline phosphatase

    c. creatinine phosphokinase

    d. lactic acid dehydrogenase

33. Anabolism is characterized by:

●   a. synthesis and storage of cell constituents

    b. breakdown of complex molecules for use in energy production

    c. digestion of foodstuffs

    d. release of cellular energy from nutrients

34. Glycogenolysis refers to:

    a. breakdown of glucose into glycogen

    b. glycogen synthesis from glucose

●   c. glycogen breakdown into glucose

    d. synthesis of glucose from amino acids and other precursors

35. Each gram of fat provides:

    a. 1 calories

    b. 4 calories

    c. 5 calories

●   d. 9 calories

36. The fat soluble vitamins are:

    a. riboflavin, niacin, vitamin C, and vitamin B12

●   b. vitamin A, vitamin D, vitamin E, vitamin K

    c. vitamin B_6, vitamin C, and folacin

    d. thiamine, vitamin A, vitamin C, and niacin

37. The diagnosis of upper or lower body obesity is established by:

    a. dividing the weight (kg) by height (cm)
 • b. dividing the waist by hip circumference
    c. by using the Metropolitan Life Insurance Tables
    d. by dividing the actual weight by desirable weight and multiplying by 100

38. Which type of obesity poses the greatest health risk in terms of heart disease, stroke, diabetes mellitus, and other health problems

 • a. upper body obesity
    b. lower body obesity

39. Malnutrition due to deficiency of both calories and protein is referred to as:

 • a. marasmus
    b. kwashirorkor
    c. bulimia
    d. cachexia

40. Complications of bulimia include:

 • a. periodontal disease, esophagitis, and dysphagia
    b. loss of appetite and anorexia
    c. constipation and cold intolerance
    d. delayed stomach emptying and abdominal distention

41. Hormones exert their action by:

    a. changing the composition of the intracellular fluid
    b. changing the composition of the extracellular fluid
 • c. interacting with specific cell receptors
    d. producing changes in the electrical potentials of target cells

42. A characteristic common to all hormones is that:

 • a. they exert their effects by altering the rate of a body reaction
    b. they are secreted at a uniform rate
    c. they must be produced in large quantities to exert their effects
    d. they always exerts their actions at the site of secretion

43. Which of the following hormones rely on protein carriers for transport in the blood stream:

 • a. steroid and thyroid hormones
    b. dopamine and epinephrine
    c. insulin and glucagon
    d. parathyroid hormone and calcitonin

44. Hormones from the anterior pituitary gland control levels of:

 • a. growth hormone, thyroid hormone, adrenal cortical hormones, and sex hormones
    b. oxytocin and antidiuretic hormone
    c. gastrin, secretin, and cholecystokinin
    d. dopamine, epinephrine, and norepinephrine

45. The concept of negative feedback regulation of hormone levels implies that:

 • a. increased hormone levels will lead to decreased hormone synthesis and release
    b. increased hormone levels will lead to increased hormone synthesis and release
    c. decreased hormone levels will lead to decreased hormone synthesis and release
    d. a change in hormone levels will have no effect on hormone synthesis and release

46. A primary disorder of adrenal cortical function is one that involves the:

    a. the hypothalamus
    b. the pituitary
    c. the target organs
    • d. adrenal cortex

47. The function/s of Growth hormone include:

    • a. growth of cartilage, bone, other tissues, and regulation of metabolic activities
    b. bone growth only
    c. the selective control of protein synthesis
    d. childhood bone growth and regulation of blood glucose levels

48. Which of the following serve to stimulate an increase in growth hormone levels:

    • a. hypoglycemia, fasting and starvation, and trauma
    b. increased glucose levels and obesity
    c. free fatty acid release and cortisol
    d. severe emotional deprivation in children

49. The term constitutional short stature describes a child with short stature due to:

    a. to psychosocial factors
    b. to malnutrition
    c. endocrine disorders
    • d. genetic influences

50. Gigantism differs from acromegaly in terms of:

    a. level of attained height
    • b. age of onset
    c. presence of accompanying metabolic derangements
    d. level of growth hormone excess that is present

51. The function of the thyroid hormone can be be described in terms of:

    a. mineral metabolism
    b. anabolic activities
    • c. metabolic rate of all body cells
    d. bone growth

52. The most profound effect of hyposecretion of thyroid hormone in the infant is:

    a. exopthalamus
    b. stridor
    • c. mental retardation
    d. goiter

53. Graves disease involves:

    a. manifestations of hypothyroidism and myxedema
    • b. hyperthyroidism, goiter, and exopthalmos
    c. hyperthyroidism and goiter
    d. a condition of severe hyperthyroidism

54. Alterations in the genitalia of children with adrenogenital syndrome result from:

    a. stimulation of genitalia growth due to excessive levels of glucocorticoids
    • b. adrenal hyperplasia and increased adrenal androgens resulting from a defect in cortisol synthesis
    c. alterations in the sex chromosomes
    d. congenital defects of the gonads

55. Acute adrenal insufficiency is characterized by:

    • a. muscle weakness, nausea and vomiting, and vascular collapse
    b. hypertension and pulmonary edema due to excess fluid retention
    c. hypernatremia and hypokalemia
    d. psychological instability and extreme muscle wasting

56. Blood sugar levels reflect:

    a. only the sugar which is ingested in the diet
    b. only the sugar which is released into the blood by the liver
  • c. the sugar which is released into the blood by the liver and that which is removed by the body tissues
    d. the sugar which is ingested in the diet and that which is removed by the tissues

57. Persons with noninsulin dependent diabetes (type II) are said to be ketosis resistant because they:

    a. are unable to convert fatty acids to ketone
  • b. have sufficient insulin to prevent fat breakdown
    c. have sufficient insulin to permit glucose transport into fat cells
    d. they have insufficient fat stores

58. The glucose tolerance test:

    a. is a urine test for sugar
    b. is a blood sugar test that is done after a meal
    c. is a fasting blood sugar test
  • d. measures blood sugar following the challenge of ingesting a concentrated glucose solution

59. The somogyi phenomenon describes:

  • a. hyperglycemia resulting from counter-regulatory mechanisms associated with hypoglycemia
    b. increased blood glucose without the presence of acidosis
    c. stress induced hypoglycemia
    d. hyperglycemia induced hypoglycemia

60. The acidosis that occurs in persons with uncontrolled insulin-dependent diabetes results from:

    a. excess sugar in the blood
  • b. ketone bodies in the blood
    c. hypoventilation and the presence of excess carbon dioxide in the blood
    d. lactic acid in the blood

61. Symptoms of hypoglycemia include:

  • a. hunger, mental confusion, and diaphoresis,
    b. flushed skin and dehydration
    c. rapid respirations and fruity smelling breath
    d. tachycardia and polyuria

62. The signs and symptoms of hypoglycemia reflect the fact that:

    a. muscle cells need glucose for normal function
  • b. glucose is the only source of energy for nervous tissue
    c. hypoglycemia decreases cerebral blood flow
    d. hypoglycemia inhibits the release of release of counter-regulatory hormones such as the catecholamines

63. The chronic complications of diabetes occur in tissues that:

    a. require insulin for transport across the cell membrane
  • b. do not require insulin for transport across the cell membrane

64. The inability to reduce insulin levels during strenuous exercise in persons with insulin-dependent diabetes can result in:

- • a. suppression of glucose release from the liver into the bloodstream and hypoglycemia
  b. decreased peripheral utilization of glucose and hyperglycemia
  c. increased lipolysis and ketoacidosis
  d. increased release of glucose from the liver into the bloodstream and hyperglycemia

65. The main effects of diabetic retinopathy include:

- a. pressure on the optic nerve
- • b. formation of new fragile retinal blood vessels
  c. changes in the shape of the lens
  d. increased production of aqueous humor

66. The reason that infections often cause ketoacidosis in persons with insulin dependent diabetes is because:

- a. infections increase metabolism and glucose requirements
- • b. the stress associated with infections increase levels of counter-regulatory hormone levels that impair diabetic control
  c. dehydration associated with infections causes blood glucose levels to become more concentrated
  d. persons tend to be more lax with their diet and insulin regimes when they are sick

67. Kussmaul breathing, which is often observed in persons with ketoacidosis, can be viewed as a compensatory mechanism in which the increased ventilation attempts to:

- a. increase the oxygen content of blood in an effort to burn the excess glucose
- • b. blow off excess carbon dioxide in an effort to increase pH
  c. increase the respiratory loss of ketone bodies as a means of controlling pH
  d. increase the oxygen supply to the brain

68. Patients with nonketotic hyperosmolalar coma suffer from:

- • a. extreme hyperglycemia and increased serum osmolality
  b. water intoxication and swelling of nerve cells
  c. extreme hyperglycemia and ketoacidosis

Alterations in Neuromuscular Function

The nervous system, in coordination with the endocrine system, provides the means for all of the integrative aspects of life. It controls not only skeletal muscle movement, but the activity of cardiac and visceral smooth muscle as well. The nervous system makes possible the reception, integration, and perception of sensory information; it provides for memory and problem solving; and it facilitates the adjustment to an ever-changing environment. This unit is organized according to physiologic function. Chapter 46 focuses on the basic organization and function of the nervous system; Chapter 47, somatosensory function and pain; Chapter 48, normal and altered autonomic nervous system function; Chapter 49, alterations in motor function; Chapter 50, disorders of brain function; Chapter 51, the eye and alterations in vision; Chapter 51, alterations in hearing and vestibular function; and Chapter 53 degenerative, demyelinating, and neoplastic disorders of the nervous system. In an effort to contain chapter size and organize content in a manner that facilitates understanding, the placement of some content has been arbitrary. For example, the discussion of multiple sclerosis and Parkinson's disease have been placed in Chapter 53 even though both disorders produce movement disorders. Likewise, the main discussion of stroke was placed in Chapter 50. A discussion of muscle tissue and membrane potentials is included in Chapter 1.

Chapter 47

Organization and Control of Neural Function

Chapter 46 provides the reader with an overview of the organization and control of neural function. The chapter begins with a discussion of the embryonic development of the nervous system, its segmental organization, and afferent and efferent pathways that connect with the various somatic and visceral structures of the body. Considerable emphasis is placed on the terminology needed to understand the nervous system and content in subsequent chapters of this unit. The chapter ends with a discussion of nerve cell communication and messenger molecules.

Teaching strategies

—Overhead transparency

Figure 47-7 shows a typical afferent and efferent neuron.

—Glossary terms

afferent	axodendritic synapse
archi layer	axon
astroglia	axosomatic synapse
axoaxonic synapse	body wall

caudal

central nervous system

cephalic

collateral pathways

conduction

dendrite

distal

dorsal and dorsal horn

dorsal root ganglia

efferent

endoneurium

epineurium

excitatory postsynaptic potential

fascicles

gamma-aminobutyric acid (GABA)

ganglia

glia

gliosis

gray matter

hierarchy of control

inhibitory postsynaptic potential

input association neuron

internuncial neurons

lateral

medial

microglia

myelin sheath

neo layer

neural crest

neuromodulators

neuron

neurotransmitters

nodes of Ranvier

oligodendroglial cells

output association neurons

paleo layer

perineurium

peripheral nervous system

postsynaptic

presynaptic

proprioception

proximal

reflex

reticular formation

reuptake

rostral

saltatory conduction

soma

spatial summation

spinothalamic tract

supporting cells

synapse

synaptic vesicles

temporal summation

tract

ventral and ventral horn

viscera

white matter

Chapter 48

Somatosensory Function and Pain

Chapter 48 is divided into two sections: the first focuses on the organization and function of the somatosensory system and the second on pain. The chapter begins with a description of somatosensory modalities, the peripheral distribution of sensory neurons (dermatomes), ascending pathways, the central distribution of sensory information, and clinical assessment of somesthetic function. The section on pain is extensively developed to include a discussion of pain mechanisms, acute and chronic pain, age factors, head pain, assessment of pain, and treatment modalities.

Teaching strategies

—Overhead transparencies

Figure 48-3 illustrates the discriminative pathway.

Figure 48-7 illustrates primary pain pathways.

—Glossary terms

A-delta fibers

acupuncture

acupressure

agonist

antagonist

agonist-antagonist

allodynia

analgesia

anesthesia

anterolateral pathway

athermia

C fibers

causalgia

cordotomy

dermatome

discriminative pathway

dorsal horn

endorphins

enkephalins

epidural

flexor-withdrawal reflex

gate control theory

guarding

herpes zoster

hypesthesia

hypothermia

hypophysectomy

intrathecal

kinesthesia

narcotic analgesic

neospinothalamic tract

neuralgia

neuropeptide

nociception

opioids

pain perception

pain threshold

pain tolerance

paleospinothalamic tract

pattern theory

periaqueductal gray region

phantom-limb pain

placebo

primary sensory cortex

proprioception

referred pain

rhizotomy

shingles

sensory unit

somesthetic

sensory modality

specificity theory

stimulation-induced analgesia

substance P

tactile

tic douloureaux

tolerance

transcutaneous electrical nerve stimulation (TENS)

visceral pain

—Other teaching strategies

Have students design a pain assessment tool for a specific age group such as an infant or child.

Chapter 49

Normal and Altered Autonomic Nervous System Function

The ability to maintain homeostasis and perform the activities of daily living in an ever changing physical environment is largely vested in the autonomic nervous system. Chapter 48 is divided into two parts: (1) the organization and control of the autonomic nervous system (ANS), and (2) disorders of the ANS. Additional content on ANS function as it relates to specific body systems is integrated into other chapters of the book.

Teaching strategies

—Glossary terms

acetylcholine

aceylcholinesterase

adrenergic receptors

alpha1 and alpha2 receptors

anhidrosis

anticholinergic

antimuscarinic

Argyll Robertson pupil

beta1 and beta2 receptors

catecholamines

cholinergic	ganglion	orthostatic (postural) hypotension	respiratory sinus arrhythmia
cranial nerves	Hirschsprung's disease	parasympathetic	reuptake
denervation hypersensitivity	Horner's syndrome	pheochromocytoma	sympathetic
dopamine	hyperhidrosis	postganglionic	syncope
endogenous neuromediators	muscarinic receptors	preganglionic	vagus
epinephrine	nicotinic receptors	progressive autonomic failure	visceral
exogenous	norepinephrine		

Chapter 50

Alterations in Motor Function

Movement in the external environment involves the coordinated function of somatosensory and motor neurons. It requires not only that muscles move but also that their movement be programmed in a manner that provides for smooth and coordinated movement. Chapter 49 is organized into five sections: (1) control of motor function, (2) disorders of the neuromuscular unit, (3) alterations in muscle tone and motor power, (4) alterations in movement coordination and abnormal movements, and (5) spinal cord injury.

Teaching strategies

—Overhead transparencies

Figure 50-1 diagrams the neural pathways for control of motor function.

Figure 50-13 shows the structure of the three types of vertebrae: (1) cervical, (2) thoracic, and (3) lumbar. This figure is intended to help students visualize the vertebral structures and the location of the spinal cord, vertebral artery, vertebral vein, and sympathetic nerves.

—Glossary terms

abductors

adductors

agonists

antagonists

ataxia

atrophy

autonomic hyperreflexia

Babinski's sign

ballismus

brain stem

carpal tunnel syndrome

cauda equina

choreiform

clonus

compression injury

corticospinal tract

dystonia

extensors

extrapyramidal system

fasciculations

fibrillations

flaccid paralysis

flexors

Guillain-Barré syndrome

hemiballismus

hemiparesis

hyperkinesia

lower motoneuron

monoparesis

motoneuron

motor cortex

motor end-plate

muscular dystrophy

myasthenia gravis

myotatic reflex

neuromuscular junction

muscle spindles

muscle tone

paresis

paralysis

paraplegia

pia mater

polyneuropathies

pronation

pyramidal system

quadriplegia

segmental spinal
nerves

spastic paralysis

supination

supplementary
motor cortex

synergists

tetany

upper motoneuron

vasovagal response

Wallerian
degeneration

Chapter 51

Disorders of Brain Function

Chapter 51 focuses on disorders of brain function. The chapter content includes: (1) a review of normal brain structure and function; (2) alterations in cerebral blood flow, including hypoxic and ischemic brain injury, cerebral vascular accident, and cerebral aneurysms and subarachnoid hemorrhage; (3) alterations in cerebral volume and pressure; (4) brain injury and infection, (5) altered levels of consciousness and brain death; and (6) seizure disorders.

Teaching strategies

—Overhead transparencies

Figure 51-3 shows a midsagittal section of the brain.

Figure 51-11 shows the flow of cerebrospinal fluid from the time of its formation in the choroid plexus until its return to the blood in the superior sagittal sinus.

—Glossary terms

aura

abducent nerve

anterior cerebral
artery

arachnoid

arachnoid villi

brain death

brain herniation

blood-brain barrier

brain scan

Brudzinski's sign

cerebellum

cerebral dominance

cerebral
hemispheres

cerebral perfusion
pressure

cerebral vascular
accident

choroid plexus

circle of Willis

common carotid

concussion

contusion

coup/contrecoup
injury

cytotoxic edema

diencephalon

dura

external carotid
artery

encephalitis

epilepsy

extravasation

facial nerve

falx cerebri

forebrain

frontal lobe

glossopharyngeal
nerve

infratentorial

hemiattention and
hemineglect

hindbrain

hydrocephalus

hypoglossal nerve

internal capsule

internal carotid
artery

Kernig's sign

limbic lobe

meninges

metaencephalon

medulla

meningitis

midbrain

middle cerebral
artery

Monro-Kellie
hypothesis

no-reflow
phenomenon

nuchal rigidity

occipital lobe

oculomotor nerve

pia mater

parietal lobe

photophobia

pons

posterior cerebral
artery

positron emission
tomography (PET)

premotor cortex

temporal lobe

transient ischemic
attacks

sagittal sinus

seizure

stroke (embolic,
thrombotic,
lacunar infarcts)

subdural space

subarachnoid space

subarachnoid
hemorrhage

supratentorial

tentorium

trigeminal nerve

trochlear

vagus nerve

vasogenic edema

ventricular system

vertebral artery

vestibulochlear
nerve

Chapter 52

Alterations in Vision

Chapter 52 focuses on the eye and alteration in vision. The chapter is organized into six sections: (1) the eye and supporting structures, (2) intraocular pressure, (3) optics and lens function, (4) vitreous and retinal function, (5) visual pathways and cortical centers, (6) eye movements. Each section contains a description of normal and altered function.

Teaching strategies

—Glossary terms

accommodation

albinism

amblyopia

anopia

aphakia

astigmatism

blepharitis

canthus

cataract

cornea

conjugate
movements

conjunctivitis

cycloplegia

dacryocystitis

epicanthic fold

extrinsic eye muscles

fovea

glaucoma
(narrow-angle and
wide-angle)

hemianopia

heteronymous

homonymous

hordeolum (style)

horizontal gaze

hyperopia

hypertelorism

hypotelorism

keratitis

lacrimal

limbus

macula

macular
degeneration

microaneurysms

myopia

neovacularization

ophthalmoscopy

optic tremor

papilledema

photoreceptors

presbyopia

quadrantanopia

refraction

retinal detachment

retinitis pigmentosa

retinopathy

retrolental
fibroplasia

saccadic movements

Schlemm's canal

sclera

Sjogren's syndrome

strabismus

palpebrae

uveitis

vergence
movements

vertical gaze

visual fields

—Other teaching strategies

A. Arrange to have students check visual fields (p. 1001), transillumination (p. 984), pupillary reflexes (p. 987), eye movement and gaze, and the retina using an opthalmoscope.

B. Obtain various lenses and have students look through them to observe what it would be like to have an error in refraction.

Chapter 53

Alterations in Hearing and Vestibular Function

The ears are paired organs responsible for hearing and maintenance of equilibrium and effective posture. The ear consists of an external ear, middle, and inner ear. The external and middle ear function in capturing, transmitting, and amplifying sound. The inner ear contains the receptive organs that are selectively stimulated by either sound waves (hearing) or head position and motion (vesitublar function). Chapter 52 focuses on alterations in hearing and disorders of auditory function and vestibular function and disorders of vestibular function. The chapter includes a discussion of otitis media, disorders of the inner ear and deafness, nystagmus, motion sickness, and Meniere's syndrome.

Teaching Strategies
—Glossary Terms

audiogram

auricle

brain stem-evoked potentials

cholesteatoma

cochlear duct

cerumen

conductive hearing loss

eustachian tube

malleus

mastoiditis

Meniere's syndrome

nystagmus

ossicles

otitis externa

otitis media

otosclerosis

Rinne test

Romberg test

sensorineural hearing loss

vertigo

vestibular system

Weber's test

Chapter 54

Degenerative, Demyelinating, and Neoplastic Disorders of the Nervous System

Chapter 54 presents a discussion of degenerative brain disorders, multiple sclerosis a demylinating disorders of the nervous system, and brain tumors.

Teaching Strategies

—Glossary Terms

Alzheimer's disease

astrocytoma

bradykinesia

Creutzfeld-Jakob disease

dementia

dopaminergic

Huntington's chorea

Lhermitte's syndrome

neuritic plaques

neurofibrillary tangles

oligdendroglioma

Pick's disease

pill-rolling movements

sundown syndrome

Wernicke-Korakoff syndrome

Examination Questions

1. The central nervous system consists of the:

   a. the brain
   ● b. the brain and spinal cord
   c. the brain and brain stem
   d. the spinal cord and peripheral nerves

2. Afferent neurons:

   ● a. carry sensory information toward the central nervous system
   b. carry sensory information away from the central nervous system
   c. carry effector and motor information toward the central nervous system
   d. carry effector or motor information away from the central nervous system

3. Somatic nerves innervate:

   ● a. skeletal muscles and the pilomotor muscles in the skin
   b. the heart and gastrointestinal tract
   c. skeletal muscles and blood vessels
   d. skeletal muscles of the extremities and inner lining of pleura and other body cavities

4. The term rostral refers to the:

   a. posterior portion of the brain
   b. inferior portion of the brain
   ● c. the portion of the brain that is in the region of the nose and mouth
   d. top portion of the brain

5. The dorsal cell columns contain:

   ● a. sensory neurons
   b. motor neurons
   c. sympathetic motor neurons
   d. parasympathetic motor neurons

6. The spinothalamic tract travels from the:

   ● a. spinal cord to the thalamus
   b. thalamus to the spinal cord
   c. brain stem to the spinal cord
   d. spinal cord to the parietal cortex

7. Which one of the following cells is responsible for myelin formation in the CNS:

   a. Schwann cells
   ● b. oligodendroglial cells
   c. astrocytes
   d. microglial cells

8. Which one of the following statements is true as it refers to regeneration of a peripheral nerve axon:

   a. peripheral nerve axons are incapable of regeneration
   ● b. the presence of the endoneurial sheath is necessary for regeneration to occur
   c. the presence of the myelin sheath is necessary for regeneration to occur
   d. only afferent nerves are capable of regeneration

9. The major source of fuel for the nervous system is:

    a. ketones
    b. fatty acids
    • c. glucos
    d. amino acids

10. An important inhibitory neurotransmitter in the nervous system is:

    a. epinephrine
    b. dopamine
    c. acetylcholine
    • d. gamma-aminobutyric acid (GABA)

11. The autonomic nervous system is usually viewed as a:

    • a. visceral efferent system
    b. visceral afferent system
    c. visceral afferent and efferent system
    d. somatic afferent and visceral efferent system

12. The outflow of the sympathetic nervous system can be described as:

    a. thoracic
    • b. thoracolumbar
    c. cranial
    d. craniosacral

13. The neuromediator/s for postganglionic sympathetic neurons that innervate the sweat glands is:

    a. acetylcholine
    b. acetycholine and norepinephrine
    • c. norepinephrine and epinephrine
    d. dopamine

14. The major mechanism for termination of neurotransmitter action in the sympathetic nervous system is:

    a. diffusion of neurotransmitter away from the synapse
    • b. reuptake into the presynaptic neuron
    c. degradation by catechol-O-methyl-transferase (COMT)
    d. uptake and degradation in the postsynaptic neuron

15. In skeletal muscle blood vessels, stimulation of beta receptors produces:

    a. vasoconstriction
    • b. vasodilation

16. In the eye, the anticholinergic drug atropine produces:

    a. pupil constriction and loss of accommodation
    • b. pupil dilatation and loss of accommodation
    c. pupil dilatation only
    d. pupil constriction only

17. Parasympathetic stimulation of the heart:

    • a. decreases heart rate
    b. increases heart rate
    c. decreases heart rate and force of contraction
    d. increases heart rate and force of contraction

18. Factors that contribute to syncope or fainting include:

    • a. bedrest, warm environment, and sudden assumption of the upright position
    b. increased vascular volume and decreased parasympathetic function
    c. cold environment and assumption of the supine position
    d. enhanced baroreceptor function due to decreased insulin release following a meal

19. In the male, erection is primarily a:

  • a. sympathetic function
    b. parasympathetic function

20. The region of the body that is supplied by pain fibers from a single pain of dorsal root ganglia is called a:

    a. plexus
  • b. dermatome
    c. reflex arc
    d. sensory unit

21. The sensation of joint movement is referred to as:

    a. proprioception
  • b. kinesthesia
    c. somesthesia
    d. agnosia

22. Stereoagnosis refers to:

    a. lack of taste discrimination
    b. inability to recognize significant sounds
  • c. ability to identify an object by feeling it
    d. inability to recognize significant objects by sight

23. The loss of crudely localized sensation on one side of the body is suggestive pathology involving the:

    a. discriminative pathway
  • b. anterolateral pathway

24. The specificity theory of pain implies that:

    a. pain receptors share ending or pathways with other somatosensory modalities and that the pattern of nerve activity is used as a signal for pain
  • b. pain stimuli use specific receptors that are not shared by other somatosensory modalities
    c. neural gating mechanisms at the segmental spinal cord level determine the interaction between pain and other somatosensory modalities
    d. pain receptors use specific motor neurons to transmit pain information

25. Pain perception and meaning occurs at the level of the:

    a. dorsal root ganglia
    b. periaqueductal gray region of the midbrain
    c. thalamus
  • d. association areas of the sensory cortex

26. The opioids are:

    a. non-narcotic drugs that act on opiate receptors in the CNS
  • b. endogenous or exogenous chemical substances with morphine-like actions that act at the level of opiate receptors in the CNS
    c. synthetic narcotics that act at the level of nonopiate receptorsin the CNS
    d. narcotic antagonists

27. The endogenous analgesic center is located in the:

    a. dorsal horn of the spinal cord
    b. limbic system
  • c. periaqueductal gray region of the midbrain
    d. rostral medulla

28. Fast, well-localized pain has its origin in the nerve endings of:

  • a. myelinated A-delta axons
    b. unmyelinated C axons

29. The sites of referred pain are determined by:

    a. associations that are made during previous pain experiences
  - b. the segmental origin of the visceral and somatic structures during embryonic development
    c. the type of noxious stimulant that is responsible for producing the pain
    d. the duration of the pain experience

30. In contrast to acute pain, chronic pain:

    a. is not true pain but is due to psychologic factors
    b. does not have a specific location that can be clearly identified
  - c. does not evoke extensive associated autonomic nervous system responses
    d. is less likely to disrupt sleep and cause depression

31. Pain that follows a non-noxious stimuli is called

  - a. allodynia
    b. paresthesia
    c. hyperesthesia
    d. dysthesia

32. One of the main actions of aspirin in terms of pain relief is:

  - a. through inhibition of prostaglandins and their effects on the inflammatory response
    b. through inhibition of pain responses on the spinal cord level
    c. through increased production of endogenous opioids
    d. relief of tension and anxiety

33. Anticonvulsant drugs are often used for relieving pain following nerve injury because of the their ability to:

    a. block opioid receptors
  - b. block spontaneous neuronal firing
    c. increase serotonin levels
    d. reduce muscle spasm

34. A motor unit consists of:

    a. a pair of abductor and adductor muscle groups
    b. a motoneuron supplying a muscle group
  - c. a motoneuron and the muscle fibers it innervates
    d. the muscle fibers with a muscle group

35. Injury to a lower motoneuron could be expected to produce:

  - a. flaccid paralysis of the innervated muscle group
    b. spastic paralysis of the innervated muscle group
    c. loss of sensation and flaccid paralysis of the innervated muscle group
    d. loss of sensation and spastic paralysis of the innervated muscle group

36. A flexor muscle is one that serves to:

    a. increase the angle of a joint
  - b. decrease the angle of a joint
    c. move a part away from the midline of the body
    d. move a part toward the midline of the body

37. The afferent neurons of the myotatic reflex transmit:

  - a. muscle stretch or tension information
    b. nociceptive information
    c. thermal information
    d. pressure and touch information

38. In terms of motor function, the cerebellum is concerned with:

    a. skill
    b. grace
  - c. temporal smoothness
    d. reflex functions

39. A lesion of the pyramidal motor system could be expected to produce:

    a. muscle rigidity and incoordination of movement
    b. loss of discrete movement
    c. abnormal postures and automatic movements
    • d. muscle weakness and loss of fine manipulative skills

40. One of the earliest manifestations of myasthenia gravis is:

    a. respiratory paralysis
    b. orthostatic hypotension and decreased autonomic nervous system responses
    • c. weakness of the eye muscles
    d. parethesias and altered sensory function

41. The drugs physostigmine and neostigmine are used in treatment of myasthenia gravis because they:

    a. increase the number of end-plate acetylcholine receptor sites
    b. increase acetylcholine synthesis
    • c. decrease the rate at which acetylcholine is inactivated
    d. block the depolarizing effects of acetylcholine on the the end-plate receptor sites

42. A herniated disk at the lower levels of the lumbar spine will tend to cause:

    a. motor paralysis from the waist down
    • b. manifestations of altered sensory and motor function in the area of the body innervated by the nerve roots
    c. localized sensory deficits in the area of the body that is supplied by the dorsal root ganglia of that segment
    d. pain, localized sensory deficits, and hyperactive reflexes along the peripheral distribution of the nerve

43. Carpal tunnel syndrome is caused by:

    a. infectious process involving the median nerve
    • b. compression injury to the median nerve
    c. injury to the dorsal root that supplies the median nerve
    d. injury to the ventral root that supplies the median nerve

44. Guillian Barre syndrome involves a:

    • a. symmetrical sensorimotor and autonomic polyneuropathy
    b. mononeuropathy
    c. symmetrical sensorimotor disorder of the upper motor neurons
    d. polyneuropathy that is confined to the autonomic nervous system

45. Disorders of movement related to cerebellar dysfunction occur on:

    • a. the same side of the body as the cerebellar lesion and occur whether the eyes are open or closed
    b. the same side of the body as the cerebellar lesion and occur only when the eyes are closed
    c. the side of the body that is opposite the cerebellar lesion and occur whether the eyes are open or closed
    d. the side of the body that is opposite the cerebellar lesion and occur only when the eyes are closed

46. A cerebellar tremor involving the hands is one in which:

    • a. back and forth movements of the fingers become worse when the target is reached
    b. there is alternating pill-rolling movements of the fingers
    c. movements of the fingers become more controlled as the target is reached
    d. tremor movements occur when the hands are not being used for skillful purposes

47. At which level of spinal cord injury is head, neck, deltoid, bicep, diaphragm, elbow, wrist, and finger control maintained:

    a. C5
    b. C6-C7
    • c. C8
    d. T1

48. Spinal shock describes:

    • a. a transient loss of somatic and autonomic reflexes below the level of injury
    b. a hypotensive state associated with the trauma of the injury
    c. a hypovolemic shock caused by blood loss associated with injury
    d. respiratory paralysis associated with spinal cord injury

49. Autonomic hyperreflexia is characterized by:

    a. muscle spasms of the upper and lower extremities
    • b. severe hypertension and bradycardia
    c. reflex emptying of the bladder and bowel
    d. severe hypotension and shock

50. In persons with S2 to S4 spinal cord injury bladder function is characterized by:

    • a. loss of detrusor muscle function, overfilling, and leakage of urine
    b. involuntary reflex emptying
    c. loss of external sphincter control while internal sphincter control is maintained
    d. small bladder size and lack of awareness of bladder filling

51. The twelfth cranial nerve contains the lower motoneurons that control:

    a. shoulder elevation
    b. the activity of gastrointestinal tract
    • c. the intrinsic and extrinsic muscles of the tongue
    d. the muscles of facial expression

52. The somatosensory cortex is located in the:

    a. frontal lobe
    • b. parietal lobe
    c. temporal lobe
    d. occipital lobe

53. Pupillary constriction is controlled at the level of the:

    a. medulla
    b. pons
    • c. midbrain
    d. diencephalon

54. Brain injury associated with a basal skull fracture would be on the:

    a. lateral side of the brain
    b. area between the sides of the brain
    • c. underside of the brain
    d. front part of the brain

55. The tentorium cerebelli is an inner:

    a. longitudinal layer of the dura that separates the cerebral hemispheres
    • b. transverse fold of the dura that separates the occipital lobe and cerebellum
    c. transverse fold of the dura that separates the midbrain and brain stem
    d. transverse fold of the dura that separates the brain stem and the spinal cord

56. The composition of the cerebrospinal fluid is similar to extracellular fluid with the exception of:

    • a. proteins
    b. sodium
    c. bicarbonate
    d. pH

57. Cerebral blood flow is largely controlled by:

    a. the sympathetic nervous system
 • b. local mechanisms
    c. the blood-brain barrier
    d. the rate of CSF secretion and reabsorption

58. Which one of the following types of CVA usually cause pure motor or sensory deficits:

    a. thrombotic
    b. embolic
 • c. lacunar infarcts
    d. intracerebral hemorrhage

59. The use of inappropriate words or jargon is a manifestation of:

 • a. expressive aphasia
    b. receptive aphasia

60. The hemiattention and hemineglect syndromes are most common in persons with a stroke that affects the:

 • a. nondominant hemisphere
    b. dominant hemisphere

61. The most common cause of subarachnoid hemorrhage is:

 • a. cerebral aneurysm
    b. trauma
    c. atherosclerosis
    d. embolus

62. Which one of the following intracranial volumes is least able to compensate for changes in intracranial pressure:

    a. cerebrospinal fluid volume
    b. blood volume
 • c. brain tissue volume

63. Hypo-osmotic states such as water intoxication are most apt to cause:

 • a. cytotoxic cerebral edema
    b. vasogenic cerebral edema

64. Pupillary dilatation with sluggish or no reaction to light is considered as an early sign of which type of brain herniation:

    a. cingulate or across the falx
 • b. uncal or lateral
    c. central or transtentorial
    d. Infratentorial

65. A concussion is a brain injury that causes:

    a. small hemorrhages and some swelling of brain tissue
 • b. momentary interruption of brain function with or without loss of consciousness
    c. tearing or shearing of brain structures
    d. bruising of the brain

66. A frequent complication of a basal skull fracture is:

 • a. leakage of CSF from the nose and ears
    b. injury to the optic nerve
    c. deafness
    d. injury to the vestibular system

67. Which type of hematoma is of arterial origin

 • a. an epidural hematoma
    b. an acute subdural hematoma
    c. a chronic subdural hematoma

68. A lucid period that is preceded by a brief period of unconsciousness and followed by rapid progression of unconsciousness is characteristic of an:

 • a. an epidural hematoma
    b. an acute subdural hematoma
    c. a chronic subdural hematoma

69. According to the modified Monroe-Kellie hypothesis, reciprocal compensation occurs between the tissue, blood, and cerebrospinal fluid volumes of the brain. Which one of these three volumes is least able to undergo a change in volume:

    a. blood
    • b. tissue
    c. cerebrospinal fluid

70. Seizures that involve both hemispheres are classified as:

    • a. general
    b. partial

71. Tonic seizure activity is characterized by:

    a. bilateral generalized contraction of the trunk muscles
    • b. rigid and violent contractions of muscles of the extremities
    c. repeated contraction and relaxation of the major muscle groups
    d. brief absence of muscle activity of the extremities

72. The complication that is of greatest concern in persons with proptosis is:

    a. optic nerve damage
    • b. corneal irritation and scaring
    c. glaucoma
    d. retinal detachment

73. Bell's palsy reflects a paralysis of cranial nerve:

    a. III
    b. IV
    c. VI
    • d. VII

74. A differentiating feature that distinguishes red eye due to glaucoma from red eye due to other causes is:

    • a. presence of a dilated pupil and cloudy cornea
    b. constricted pupil and increased sensitivity to light
    c. reddened eyelids and watery discharge
    d. ocular discomfort and dilatation of the conjunctival vessels

75. Pupillary dilatation is termed:

    • a. mydriasis
    b. miosis
    c. aniscocoria
    d. presbyopia

76. In which type of glaucoma does prolonged pupillary dilatation produce a rise in intraocular pressure:

    • a. closed-angle
    b. open-angle

77. The chief symptom of a cataract is:

    a. the presence of halo's around lights
    • b. a decline in visual acuity
    c. loss of peripheral vision
    d. a sensation of glare

78. Dark adaptation is accompanied by an increase in:

    • a. black-gray-white vision
    b. color vision

79. The most common causes of retinal detachment are:

    • a. myopia and aphakia
    b. macular degeneration and hypertensive retinopathy
    c. retinal vein occlusion and retinitis pigmentosa
    d. presbyopia and glaucoma

80. The left lateral periphery of the visual field is seen by the:

    - a. left nasal retina
    - b. right nasal retina
    - c. left temporal retina
    - d. right temporal retina

81. Amblyopia refers to

    a. outward deviation of the eye
    b. inward deviation of the eye
    - c. diminished vision in a normally appearing eye that cannot be corrected by lenses
    d. diminished ability of the lens to accommodate to near and far vision

82. Coughing and vomiting reflexes that can occur with insertion of a speculum into the ear canal are caused by:

    - a. stimulation of vagal fibers that innervate the ear canal
    b. fear and anxiety
    c. breath holding
    d. stimulation of pain fibers in the ear canal

83. A distinguishing feature of otitis externa is:

    a. hearing impairment
    b. ear discharge
    - c. pain with movement of the external ear
    d. slight fever

84. One of the reasons that infants and small children are more susceptible to middle ear infections as compared to older children and adults is related to the fact that:

    - a. the auditory tube of infants and small children is shorter and in a more horizontal position in infants and small children
    b. the auditory tube of infants and small children is lined with a mucous membrane that is continuous with the nasopharynx
    c. there is an opening between the auditory canal and nasopharynx in infants and small children
    d. air from the nasopharynx enters the auditory tube in infants and small children

85. One of the most common complications of otitis media is:

    - a. a temporary conductive hearing loss
    b. perforation of the tympanic membrane
    c. mastoiditis
    d. cholesteatoma

86. Early hearing loss in persons with otosclerosis is characterized by:

    - a. loss of the ability to hear a whisper or someone speaking at distance
    b. inability to hear their own voice
    c. difficulty hearing in a noisy environment
    d. inability to hear on the telephone

87. One of the causes of conductive hearing loss is:

    a. a lesion of the auditory nerve
    b. disease of the inner ear
    - c. impacted ear wax
    d. effect of an ototoxic drug

88. The Weber's test is used to evaluate:

• a. bone conduction
   b. air and bone conduction
   c. sensorineural hearing loss
   d. both conduction and sensorineural hearing loss

89. Nystagmus is characterized by:

   a. abnormal jerking-type eye movements
• b. normal vestibular-controlled eye movements that occur in response to head motion
   c. abnormal outward eye movements that occur in response to head motion
   d. abnormal inward eye movements that occur in response to head motion

90. Vertigo refers to:

   a. dizziness
• b. hallucinations of motion
   c. fainting
   d. light-headedness

91. The symptoms of Meniere's syndrome are caused by:

   a. destruction of the vestibulocochlear nerve
• b. overaccumulation of fluid in the semicircular ducts
   c. injury to the vestibular organs of the inner ear
   d. inflammation of the middle ear

92. Degenerative brain disorders:

   a. affect a single hemisphere of the brain
• b. affect one or more functional systems while sparing others
   c. involve a discrete local area of the brain
   d. are limited to the cortical functions of the brain

93. A major characteristic of dementia is:

• a. impairment of short- and long-term memory
   b. hallucinations
   c. uncontrolled anger
   d. aphasia

94. The second stage of Alzheimer's disease is characterized by:

   a. disorientation to time and date
• b. inappropriate social behavior
   c. inability to communicate
   d. subtle personality changes

95. A diagnosis of Alzheimer's disease is dependent upon:

   a. the presence of biochemical markers in the blood
   b. results of brain imaging or CT scans
   c. performance on psychological tests
• d. elimination of other causes of dementia

96. Which one of the following types of dementia is caused by an infectious agent:

   a. Pick's disease
• b. Cruetzfeldt-Jackob's disease
   c. Huntington's disease
   d. Wernicke-Korsakoff's syndrome

97. Which one of the following movement patterns is characteristic of Parkinson's disease:

• a. pill-rolling tremor movements of the distal extremities that occurs at rest
   b. fine intentional tremors of the fingers
   c. increased associative movements such as swinging of the arms while walking
   d. increased tendency movements to terminate abruptly once they have been initiated

98. Multiple sclerosis is a disorder of:

    a. the Schwann cells and myelin of the peripheral nervous system
  • b. the oligodendriglial cells and myelin of central nervous system

99. Vomiting that occurs with brain tumors usually:

  • a. occurs without warning and is not preceded by nausea
    b. is of small volume and preceded by nausea
    c. occurs only at night and while the person is in the supine position
    d. is preceded by nausea and occurs after meals

100. Manifestations of papilledema include:

    a. red eyes and diplopia
    b. constricted pupils and decreased visual acuity
  • c. a decrease in visual acuity, diplopia, and visual field defects
    d. dilated pupils and halo's around lights

Alterations in Skeletal Support and Movement

The skeletal system provides support for attachment of muscles, tendons, and ligaments. It protects and maintains soft tissues in their proper position, maintains the body's shape, and provides the stability needed for movement in the external environment. The skeletal system also serves as a storage reservoir for calcium and phosphate, and the central cavity of some bones contains the hematopoietic connective tissue in which blood cells are formed. This unit is divided into four chapters: Chapter 55, the structure and function of the skeletal system; Chapter 56, alterations in skeletal function: trauma and infection; Chapter 57, alterations in skeletal function: congenital disorders, metabolic bone disease, and neoplasms; and Chapter 58, alterations in skeletal function: rheumatic disorders.

Chapter 55

Structure and Function of the Skeletal System

Chapter 55 provides the student with an introduction to the skeletal system. The chapter is divided into two parts: the first part focuses on the characteristics and the second on joints and articulations. It is recommended that students read this chapter in preparation for understanding the content in subsequent chapters.

Teaching strategies

—Overhead transparencies

Figure 55-3 depicts the structures of a long bone including the epiphysis, diaphysis, and metaphysis.

Figure 55-4 illustrates the structures of a diarthroidal joint.

—Glossary terms

amphiarthroses	Haversian canal
bursa	hyaline cartilage
canaliculi	lacuna
cancellous bone	ligaments
chondrocytes	matrix
compact bone	meniscus
collagen	metaphysis
diaphysis	osteoblast
diarthroses	osteoclast
endosteum	osteocyte
epiphysis	osteogenic cell
fibrocartilage	perichondrium

periosteum

synarthroses

synovium

tendons

Volkmann's canal

A. If available use a skeleton to illustrate organization and structure of the skeletal system.

Chapter 56

Alterations in Skeletal Function: Trauma and Infection

Chapter 56 focuses on alterations in skeletal function due to trauma and infection. The chapter contains content on soft tissue injury such as sprains and strains, dislocations, fractures, iatrogenic bone infections, acute and chronic osteomyelitis, and tuberculosis of the bone. A description of the compartment syndrome and fat emboli are included in the discussion of fracture complications.

Teaching strategies

—Overhead transparencies

Figure 56-2 shows the classification of fractures.

Figure 56-4 shows the healing of a fracture.

—Glossary terms

bacteremia

callus

chondromalacia

contusion

countertraction

dislocation

fractures (comminuted, compound, compression, greenstick, simple)

hematogenous

hematoma

iatrogenic

isometric

laceration

osteomyelitis

sequestrum

sprain

strain

subluxation

union

malunion

Chapter 57

Alterations in Skeletal Function: Congenital Disorders, Metabolic Bone Disease, and Neoplasms

Chapter 57 describes alterations in skeletal function due to congenital disorders, metabolic bone disease, and neoplasms. The chapter is organized into three sections: alterations in skeletal growth and development, metabolic bone disease, and neoplasms. One of the unique features of this chapter is the inclusion of normal developmental variants in muscle tone and joint function, such as toeing-in and toeing out, that occur in infants and children. The chapter also includes a discussion of skeletal disorders such as osteoporosis that occur later in life. Because of its application to bone formation and metabolism, the content on parathyroid hormone, calcitonin, and vitamin D has been included in this chapter.

Teaching strategies

—Glossary terms

calcaneovalgus

chondroblastoma

chondroma

congenital

coxa

equinovarus

genu

growth plate

ossification

osteogenesis imperfecta

osteochondroses

osteomalacia

osteopenia

osteoporosis

osteosarcoma

osteotomy

resorption

scoliosis

toeing-in

toeing-out

torsional forces

valgum

varum

—Other teaching strategies

A. Obtain photographs or slides of normal variants of joint and muscles changes that occur in infants and small children and use as part of lecture or discussion content. Include a child sitting in the M and W positions.

B. Arrange to have students participate in a scoliosis screening program.

Chapter 58

Alterations in Skeletal Function: Rheumatic Disorders

Arthritis affects persons of all age groups and is a leading cause of discomfort and impaired mobility. Chapter 57 focuses on rheumatic disorders including rheumatoid arthritis, osteoarthritis, spondylarthropathies, and crystal-induced arthropathies.

Teaching Strategies

—Overhead Transparencies

Figure 58-1 can be used to show the changes in joint structure that occur with rheumatoid arthritis.

Figure 58-5 illustrates the changes that occur with osteoarthritis. The Arthritis Foundation has additional slides that can be used in teaching content related to arthritis. The *Primer on the Rheumatic Diseases*, which is available through the Arthritis Foundation, is an excellent reference regarding rheumatic disorders.

—Glossary Terms

ankylosing

autologous

carpometacarpal

interphalangeal

hallus valgus

hyperuricemia

metacarpophalangeal

osteoarthritis

osteophyte

pannus

rheumatoid arthritis

rheumatoid factor

sacroileitis

sicca complex

Sjogren's syndrome

spondyloarthropathies

uricosuric

vasculitis

Examination questions

1. The axial skeleton consists of the bones of the:

   a. the upper and lower extremities
   - b. vertebral column, shoulders, and hips
   c. skull, vertebral column, and thorax
   d. arms and hands and those of the legs and feet

2. The periosteum is the:

   a. membrane that lines the spaces of spongy bone
   b. lining of the marrow cavities
   c. is the lining of the haversian canals of compact bone
   - d. is the outer fibrous covering of bone

3. Which one of the following types of bone cells is responsible for building bone matrix:

   a. osteoclasts
   - b. osteoblasts
   c. osteogenic cells
   d. osteocytes

4. Which one of the following serves to connect muscles to bones:

   - a. tendons
   b. ligaments
   c. bursae
   d. menisci

5. The hip joint is an example of:

   a. a synarthoidal joint
   b. a amphiarthroidal joint
   - c. an diarthrodial joint

6. Longitudinal bone growth occurs in:

   a. metaphysis
   b. diaphysis
   - c. epiphysis

7. A sprain involves:

   a. stretching injury to a muscle or musculotendinous unit
   - b. injury to the ligamentous structures that support a joint
   c. partial dislocation in which bone ends within a joint are still in partial contact with each other
   d. displacement and loss of articulation of bone ends within the joint capsule

8. A fatigue, or stress, fracture is caused by:

   a. direct force
   b. massive muscle contraction
   - c. repeated wear on a bone
   d. a disease process that weakens bone

9. A comminuted fracture is characterized by:

   a. a partial break in bone continuity
   b. injury in which two bones are crushed together
   - c. an injury in which the bone is broken into two more pieces
   d. an injury in which the bone fragments have broken through the skin

10. Which type of fracture is usually accompanied by the greatest blood loss:

    a. radius and ulna
    b. tibia and fibula
    c. femur
    • d. pelvis

11. The main reason for applying a cast with a joint in partial flexion is to prevent:

    a. muscle atrophy
    • b. rotation of the extremity within the cast
    c. deformities such as contractures and dislocations
    d. pressure on the joint surface

12. The normal sequence for bone healing is:

    a. callus formation, hematoma formation, ossification, and remodeling
    • b. hematoma formation, callus formation, ossification, and remodeling
    c. hematoma formation, callus formation, remodeling, and ossification
    d. callus formation, hematoma formation, remodeling, and ossification

13. The compartment syndrome involves:

    a. a large compartment or area of localized hemorrhage
    • b. nerve and blood vessel compression caused by swelling of tissues enclosed within muscle fascia
    c. bleeding into a joint space
    d. presence of a loose body with a joint space

14. A frequent early symptom of fat emboli is:

    a. dyspnea
    b. hypotension
    • c. disorientation or subtle change in behavior
    d. cough and dyspnea

15. The most common cause of osteomyelitis is:

    a. infection spread through the blood stream
    b. tuberculosis
    • c. direct contamination of an open wound
    d. rheumatic diseases

16. Genu varum refers to:

    • a. outward bowing of the knees
    b. decreased space between the knees
    c. internal rotation of the hip
    d. toeing-in due to adduction of the forefoot

17. Legg-Calve-Perthes disease involves:

    a. partial separation of the tibial tuberosity
    • b. avascular necrosis of bone and marrow involving the epiphysis in the femoral head
    c. slipped capital femoral epiphysis

18. Signs of congenital hip dislocation include:

    • a. asymmetry of the hip or gluteal folds
    b. lack of movement in the affected leg
    c. crying of the infant when the affected leg is moved
    d. turning in of the foot on the affected leg

19. Effective treatment of congenital dislocation of the hip is most effective if it is initiated before the child:

    a. begins to roll from side to side
    • b. begins to stand or bear weight on the hip
    c. begins to run and use the hip for more complicated motions such as riding a tricycle
    d. reaches adolescence and epiphyseal closure occurs

20. In contrast to structural scoliosis, postural scoliosis:

    a. only occurs in male children
    • b. corrects with bending
    c. occurs mainly in adolescent girls
    d. causes a curve in the thoracic area that is convex and to the left

21. Osteogenesis imperfecta is a genetic disorder characterized by defective:

    • a. synthesis of connective tissue and bone matrix
    b. osteoclast activity and bone resorption
    c. osteoblast activity and bone formation
    d. mineralization of bone matrix

22. Calcitonin functions in:

    a. release of calcium from bone
    b. conservation of calcium by the kidney
    c. enhanced absorption of calcium from the gastrointestinal tract
    • d. inhibiting the release of calcium from bone

23. The <u>final step</u> in the Vitamin D activation occurs in the:

    a. skin
    b. gastrointestinal tract
    c. liver
    • d. kidneys

24. Osteoporosis is evidenced by:

    • a. loss of trabeculae from cancellous bone and thinning of the outer compact cortical bone
    b. inadequate mineralization of the organic bone matrix
    c. formation of sclerotic and osteoblastic bone lesions
    d. impaired synthesis of the organic matrix of bone

25. Osteomalacia causes:

    a. loss of bone matrix and brittle bones
    • b. inadequate mineralization and softening of bones

26. Which one of the following conditions predisposes to the development of osteomalacia:

    a. corticosteroid therapy
    b. lack of dietary calcium
    c. menopause
    • d. increased renal phosphorus losses

27. The major symptoms of bone cancer are:

    • a. persistant pain that becomes worse at night, unexplained swelling over a bone, increased skin warmth over a bone
    b. a limp that is relieved by rest and skin discoloration over a bone
    c. unexplained swelling, lack of sensation, and coolness over a bone
    d. general swelling over a bone, fever, and decreased arterial pulsations

28. The joint that is most commonly affected in rheumatoid arthritis is the:

    a. hip
    b. ankle
    c. wrist
    • d. knee

29. The pathologic changes that occur in rheumatoid arthritis begin with:

    • a. destructive hyperplasia of the synovial membrane and subsynovial tissues
    b. destruction and loss of the articular cartilage and subchondral bone
    c. inflammation at the sites where ligaments insert into bone
    d. softening of the articular cartilage

30. In a person with rheumatoid arthritis of the knees, the bulge sign is used to detect the presence of:

    • a. excess synovial fluid
    b. an enlarged bursae behind the knee
    c. a genu valgus deformity
    d. joint instability caused by quadriceps atrophy

31. Diagnosis of rheumatoid arthritis is based on:

• a. symmetrical joint swelling, morning stiffness, and the presence of rheumatoid nodules

   b. pain that increases throughout the day, limitation of motion, and presence of crepitus sounds when the joint is moved

   c. persistent or intermittent back pain with prolonged stiffness

   d. fever and signs of a systemic inflammatory response, hard and warm swollen joints, and stiffness that becomes worse following joint use

32. The rationale for including physical rest in the treatment plan of a person with rheumatoid arthritis is to:

• a. reduce joint stress and relieve pain

   b. maintain joint function and muscle strength

   c. suppress the inflammatory process and relieve pain

   d. reduce swelling and stiffness

33. The signs and symptoms of Sjogren's syndrome include:

   a. low-grade fever, fatigue, and weakness

• b. dryness of the mouth and eyes due to reduced lacrimal and salivary gland secretions

   c. chest pain and pleural friction rub

   d. visual disturbances due to inflammation of the sclera and episclera

34. The form of juvenile rheumatoid arthritis that is called Still's disease is characterized by:

• a. an onset of daily intermittent high fever and other systemic manifestations

   b. antinuclear antibodies and the presence of sacroilitis and arthritis of the lower extremities

   c. an onset of polyarticular disease resembling the adult form of the disease

   d. seronegative arthritis with asymmetric arthritis of the toes and fingers

35. Schober's sign is used to determine the:

   a. the extent of hip flexion

   b. knee movement

• c. lumbar spine flexion

   d. wrist movement

36. The LE factor that is found in the blood of persons with systemic lupus erythematosus is:

• a. an anti-DNA antibody

   b. a defective white blood cell

   c. an abnormal macrophage

   d. a T4 lymphocyte

37. The reason that persons with systemic lupus erythematosus are instructed to avoid sunlight is because sunlight:

   a. increases the risk of skin cancer

   b. increases their vitamin D level

• c. increases the severity of skin lesions on the nose and cheeks

   d. alters the circadian rhythm and impairs the immune response

Table of Transparencies

Centrioles

Mitochondrion

Chromatin

Endoplasmic reticulum

Ribosomes

Protein
Lipid — Cell
Protein — membrane

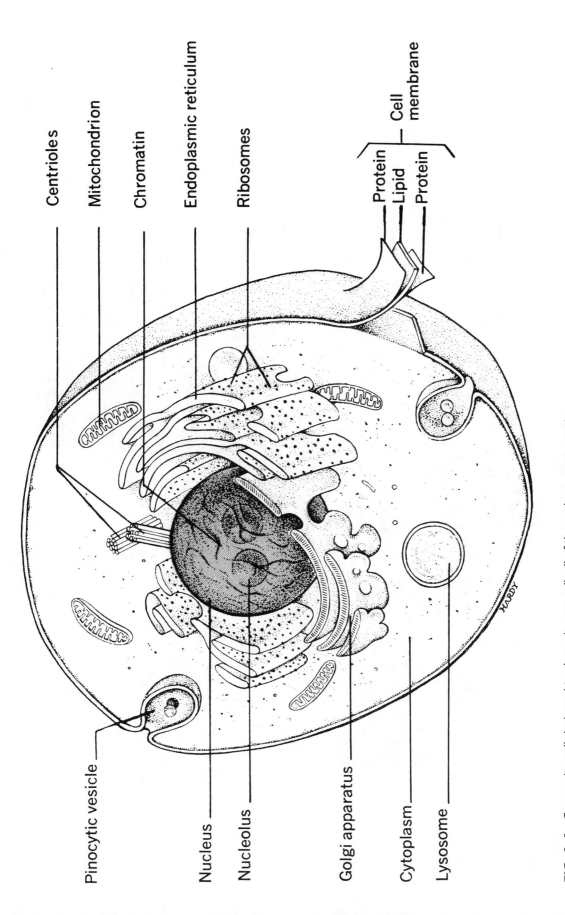

Pinocytic vesicle

Nucleus

Nucleolus

Golgi apparatus

Cytoplasm

Lysosome

HARDY

FIG. 1-1. Composite cell designed to show, in one cell, all of the various components of the nucleus and cytoplasm

Porth: Pathophysiology, 4th Edition
Copyright © 1994, J.B. Lippincott Company

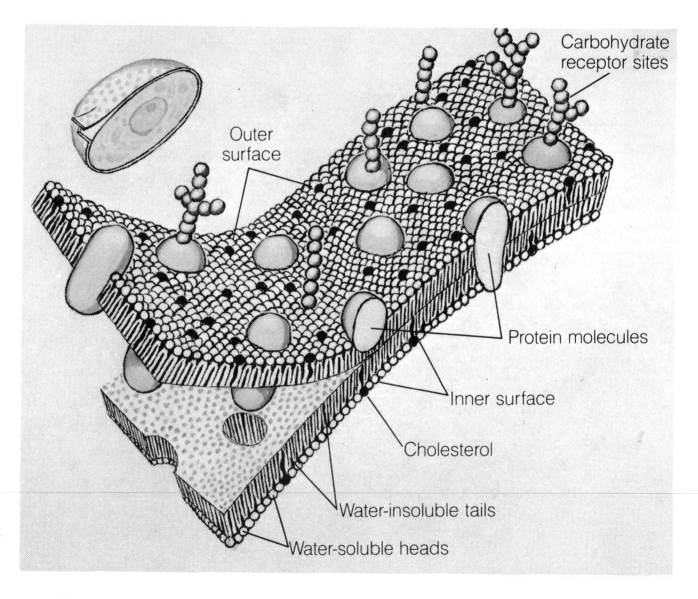

Outer
surface

Carbohydrate
receptor sites

Protein molecules

Inner surface

Cholesterol

Water-insoluble tails

Water-soluble heads

FIG. 1–6. Cell membrane. The right end is intact, but the left end has been split along
the plane of the lipid tails
Porth: Pathophysiology, 4th Edition
Copyright © 1994, J.B. Lippincott Company

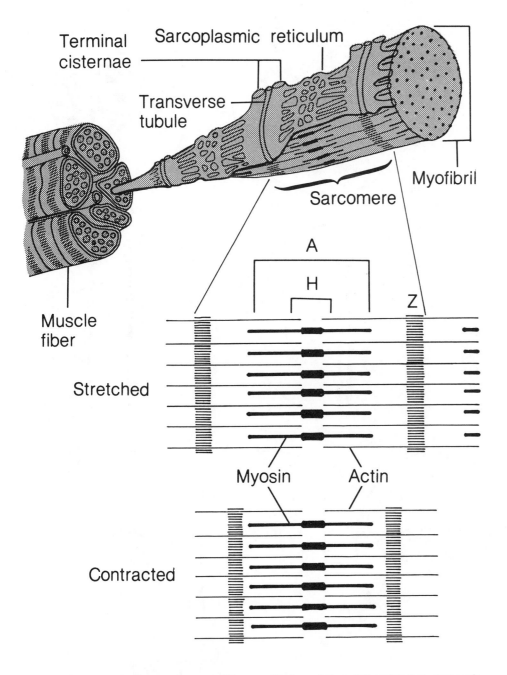

FIG. 1–20. Muscle fiber, structures of the myofibril, and the relationship between actin and myosin filaments when the muscle is stretched or contracted
Porth: Pathophysiology, 4th Edition
Copyright © 1994, J.B. Lippincott Company

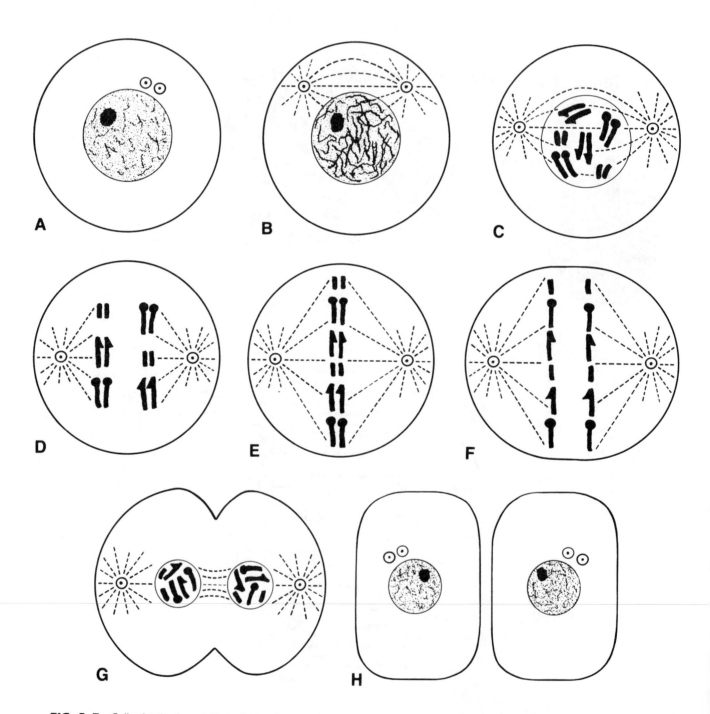

FIG. 3–7. Cell mitosis. A and H represent the nondividing cell; B, C, and D represent prophase; E represents anaphase; and G represents telophase

Porth: Pathophysiology, 4th Edition

Copyright © 1994, J.B. Lippincott Company

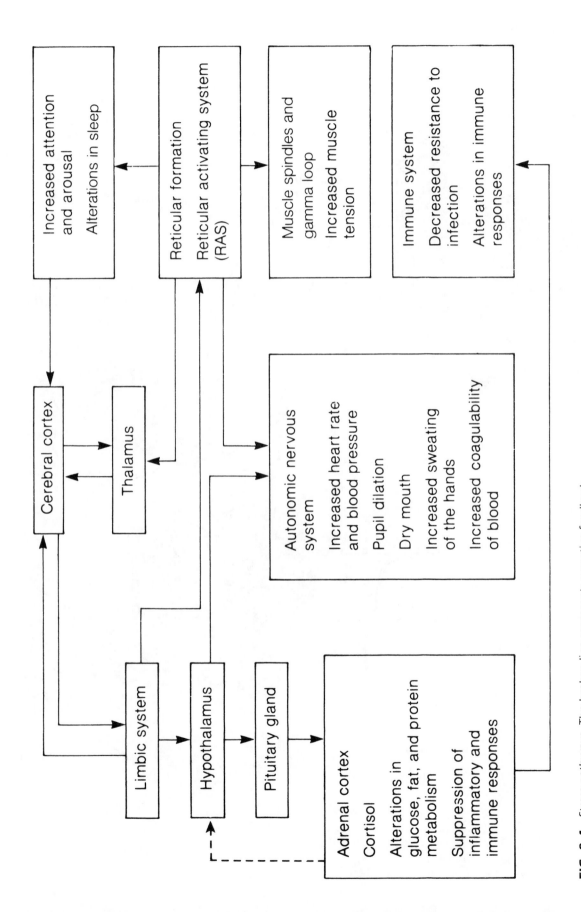

FIG. 8-1. Stress pathways. The broken line represents negative feedback
Porth: Pathophysiology, 4th Edition
Copyright © 1994, J.B. Lippincott Company

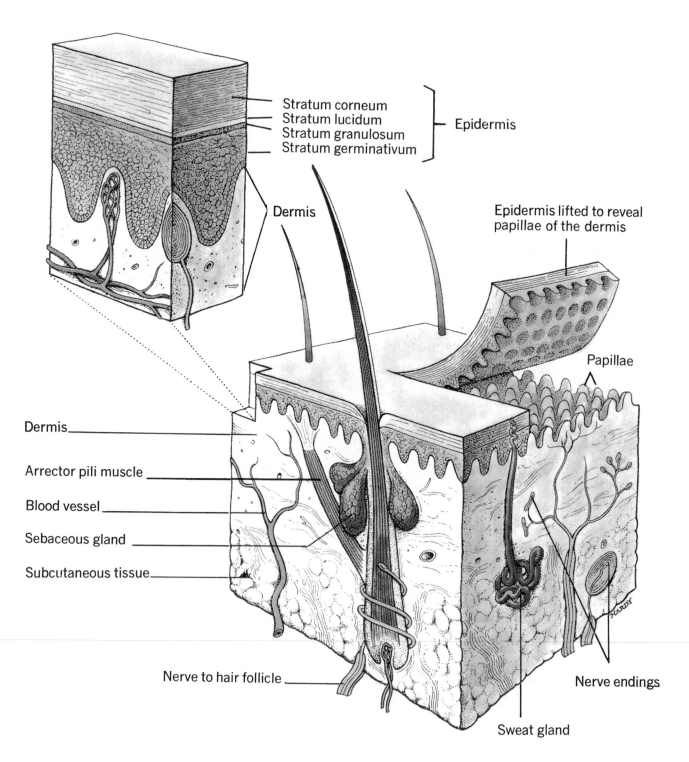

Stratum corneum
Stratum lucidum
Stratum granulosum
Stratum germinativum

Epidermis

Dermis

Epidermis lifted to reveal papillae of the dermis

Papillae

Dermis

Arrector pili muscle

Blood vessel

Sebaceous gland

Subcutaneous tissue

Nerve to hair follicle

Nerve endings

Sweat gland

FIG. 11–1. Three-dimensional view of the skin
Porth: Pathophysiology, 4th Edition
Copyright © 1994, J.B. Lippincott Company

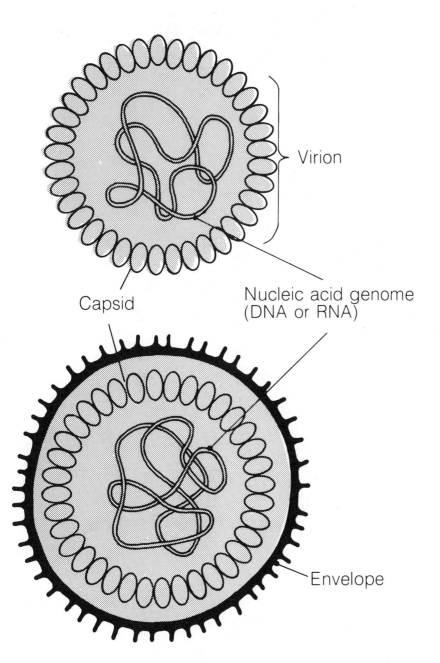

FIG. 12–1. The structure of viruses. The basic structure of a virus includes a protein coat surrounding an inner core of nucleic acid (either DNA or RNA). Some viruses may also be enclosed in a lipoprotein outer envelope

Porth: Pathophysiology, 4th Edition

Copyright © 1994, J.B. Lippincott Company

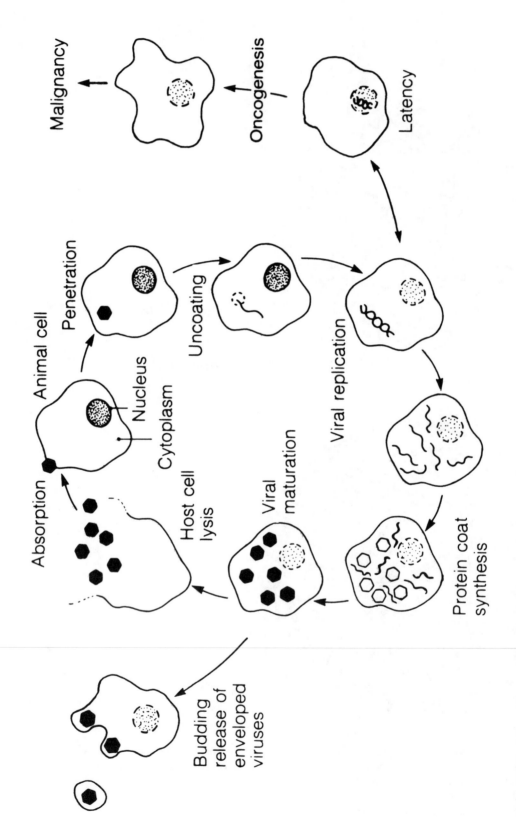

FIG. 12–2. Schematic representation of the many possible consequences of viral infection of host cells, including cell lysis (poliovirus), continuous release of budding viral particles or latency (herpesviruses) and oncogenesis (papovaviruses)
Porth: Pathophysiology. 4th Edition
Copyright © 1994, J.B. Lippincott Company

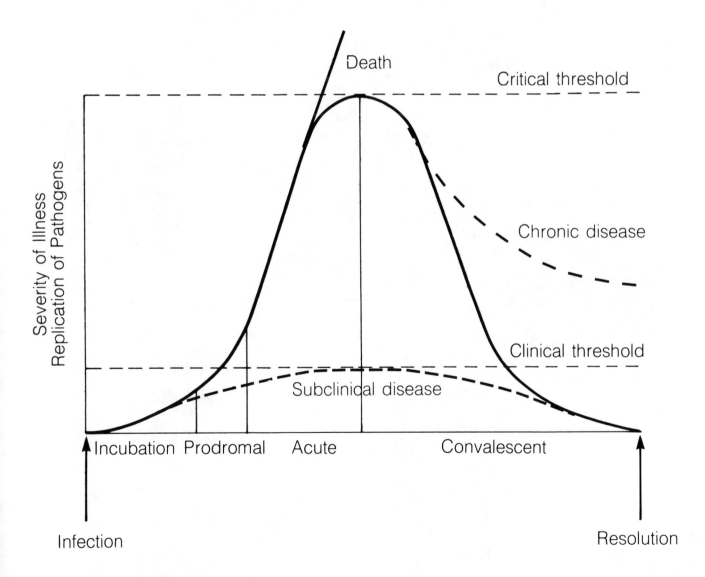

FIG. 12–5. The stages of a primary infectious disease as they appear in relation to the severity of symptoms and the numbers of infectious agents

Porth: Pathophysiology, 4th Edition
Copyright © 1994, J.B. Lippincott Company

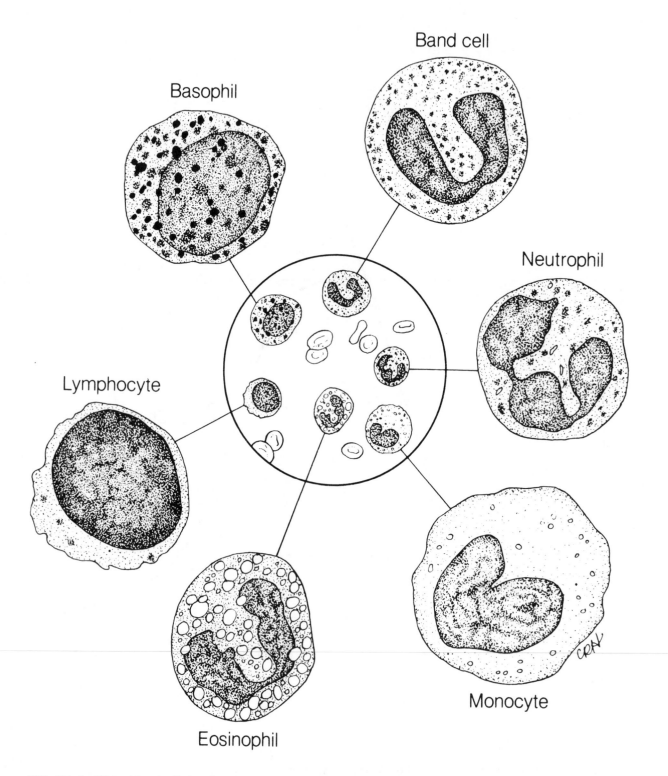

FIG. 13–1. White blood cells involved in the inflammatory response
Porth: Pathophysiology, 4th Edition
Copyright © 1994, J.B. Lippincott Company

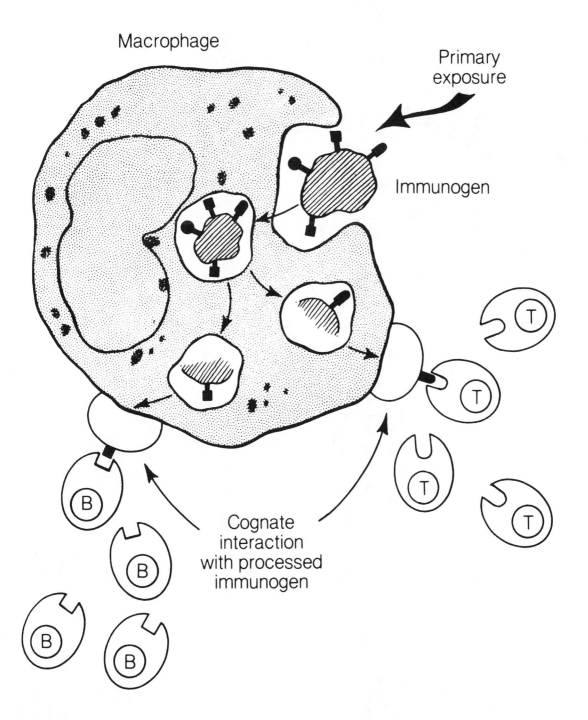

Macrophage

Primary
exposure

Immunogen

Cognate
interaction
with processed
immunogen

FIG. 13–6. The interaction between the immunogen (antigen), macrophage, and
T-lymphocytes and B-lymphocytes
Porth: Pathophysiology, 4th Edition
Copyright © 1994, J.B. Lippincott Company

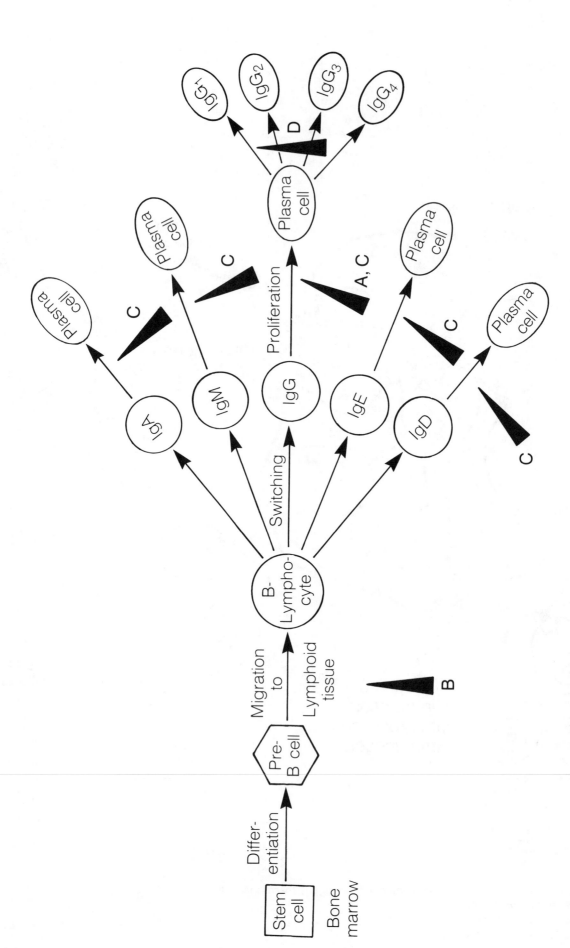

FIG. 14-1. Stem cells to mature immunoglobulin-secreting plasma cells. Arrows indicate the stage of the maturation process that is interrupted in: (A) transient hypoglobulinemia, (B) Bruton's hypogammaglobulinema, (C) common variable immunodeficiency, and (D) IgG subclass deficiency

Porth: Pathophysiology, 4th Edition

Copyright © 1994, J.B. Lippincott Company

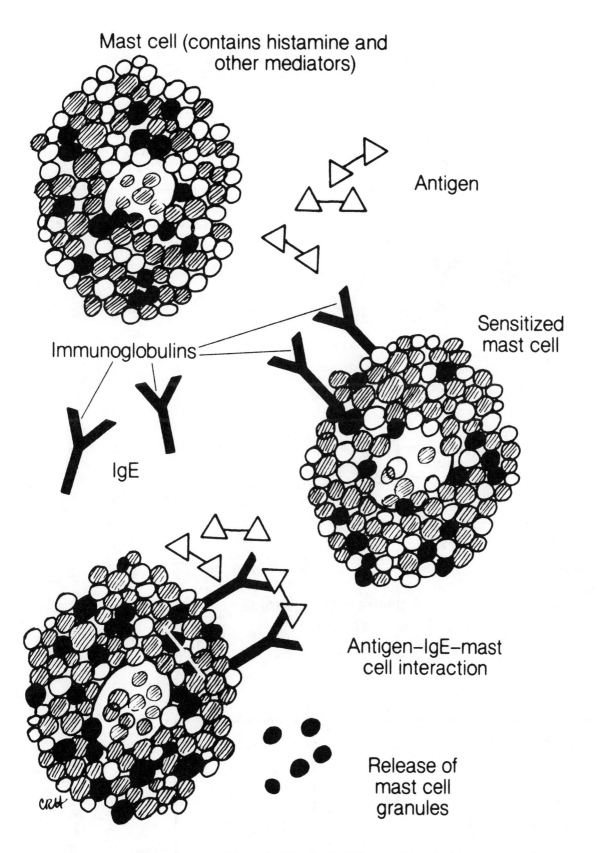

FIG. 14–4. Type I immune response that involves an allergen (antigen), immunoglobulin (IgE), and mast cell. Exposure to the allergen causes sensitization of the mast cell with subsequent binding of the allergen, which causes release of mast cell granules containing inflammatory mediators such as histamine and SRS-A

Porth: Pathophysiology, 4th Edition

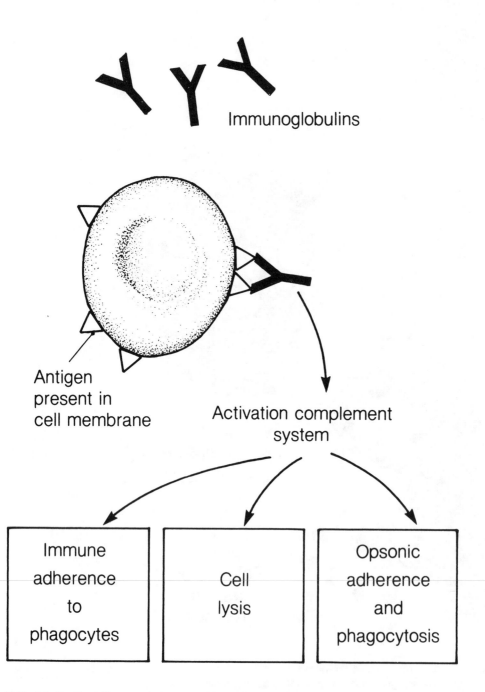

Immunoglobulins

Antigen
present in
cell membrane

Activation complement
system

| Immune adherence to phagocytes | Cell lysis | Opsonic adherence and phagocytosis |

FIG. 14–5. Type II cytotoxic immune reactions that involve immunoglobulins (IgG and IgM) and cell-surface antigens with activation of the complement system
Porth: Pathophysiology, 4th Edition
Copyright © 1994, J.B. Lippincott Company

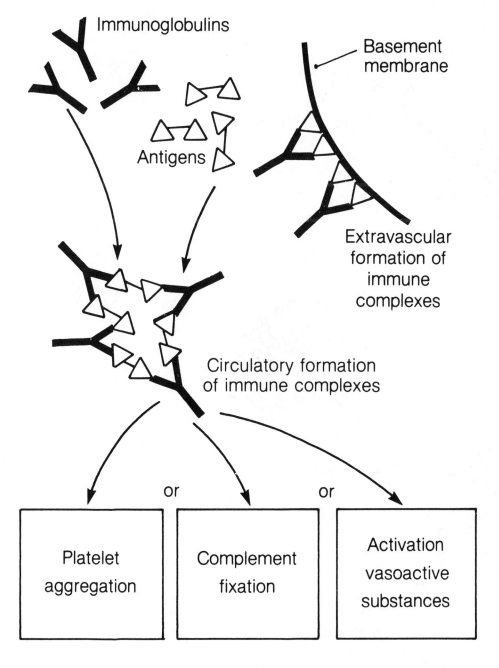

FIG. 14–6. Type III immune complex reactions that involve complement-activating IgG and IgM immunoglobulins with formation of bloodborne or extravascular immune complexes and their effects
Porth: Pathophysiology, 4th Edition
Copyright © 1994, J.B. Lippincott Company

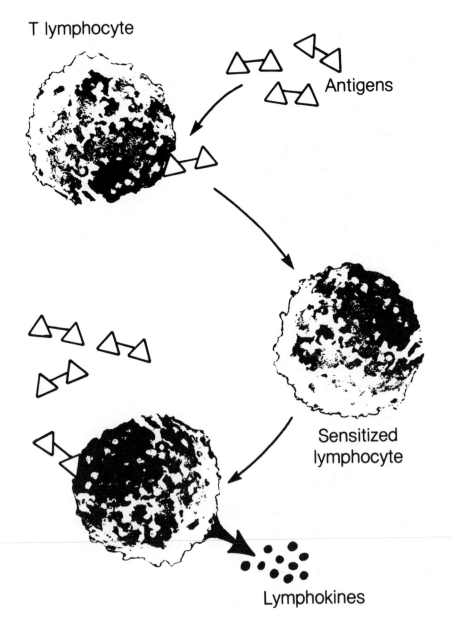

T lymphocyte

Antigens

Sensitized
lymphocyte

Lymphokines

FIG. 14–7. Type IV immune response that involves an antigen, sensitized T-lymphocyte, and lymphokines. Exposure to the antigen causes sensitization of the lymphocyte with release of lymphokines on subsequent exposures
Porth: Pathophysiology, 4th Edition
Copyright © 1994, J.B. Lippincott Company

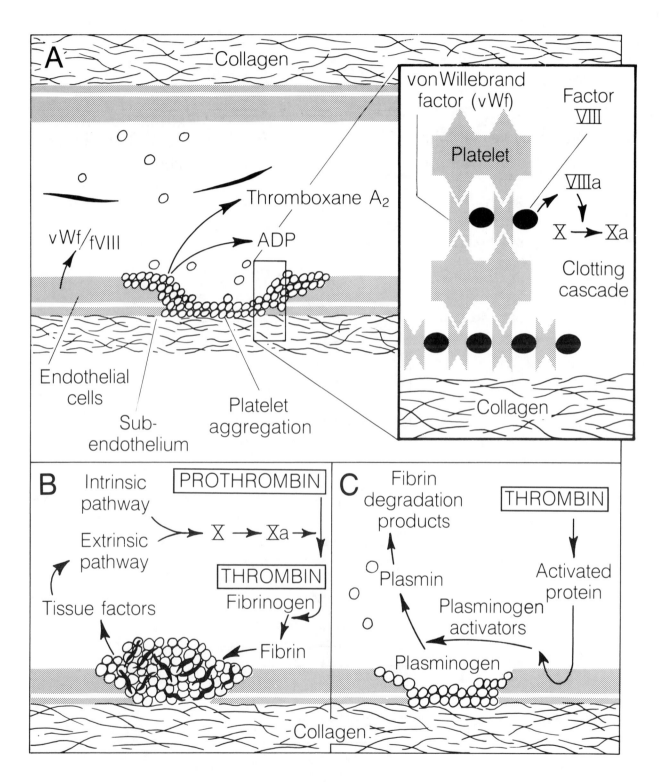

FIG. 17–1. (A) The platelet plug occurs seconds after vessel injury. (B) Coagulation factors, activated on the platelet surface, lead to the formation of thrombin and fibrin, which stabilize the platelet plug. (C) Control of the coagulation process and clot dissolution are governed by thrombin and plasminogen activators

Porth: Pathophysiology, 4th Edition

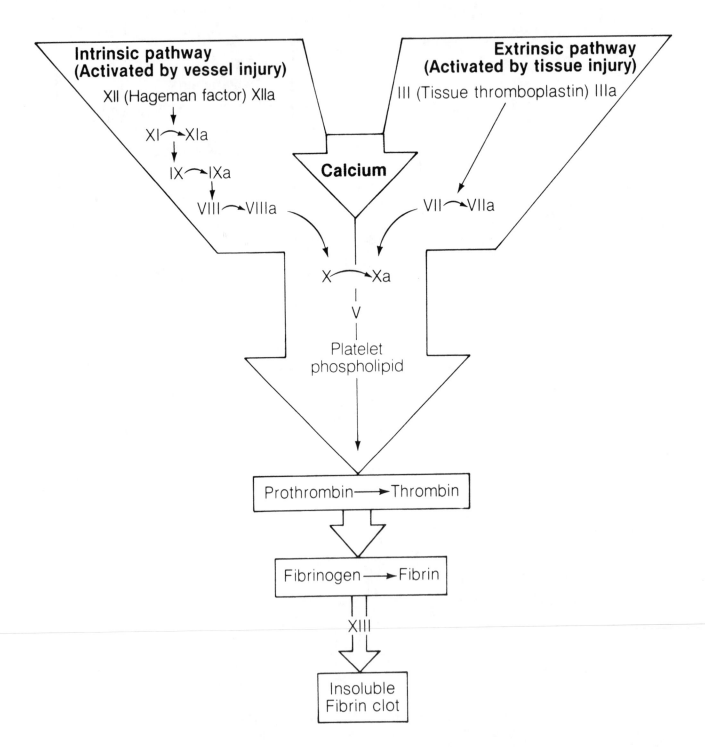

FIG. 17–3. Intrinsic and extrinsic coagulation pathways
Porth: Pathophysiology, 4th Edition
Copyright © 1994, J.B. Lippincott Company

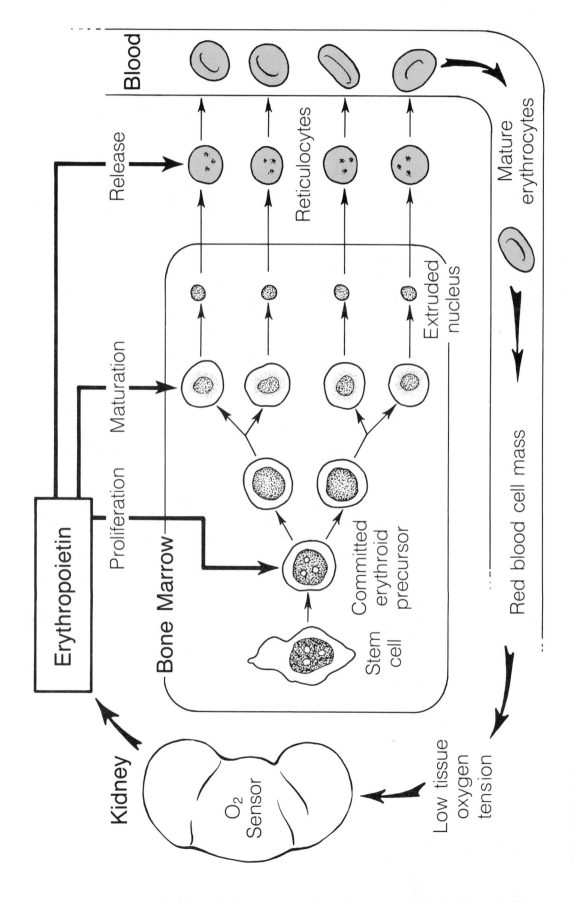

FIG. 18–3. Red blood cell development
Porth: Pathophysiology, 4th Edition
Copyright © 1994, J.B. Lippincott Company

Systemic Circulation

Pulmonary Circulation

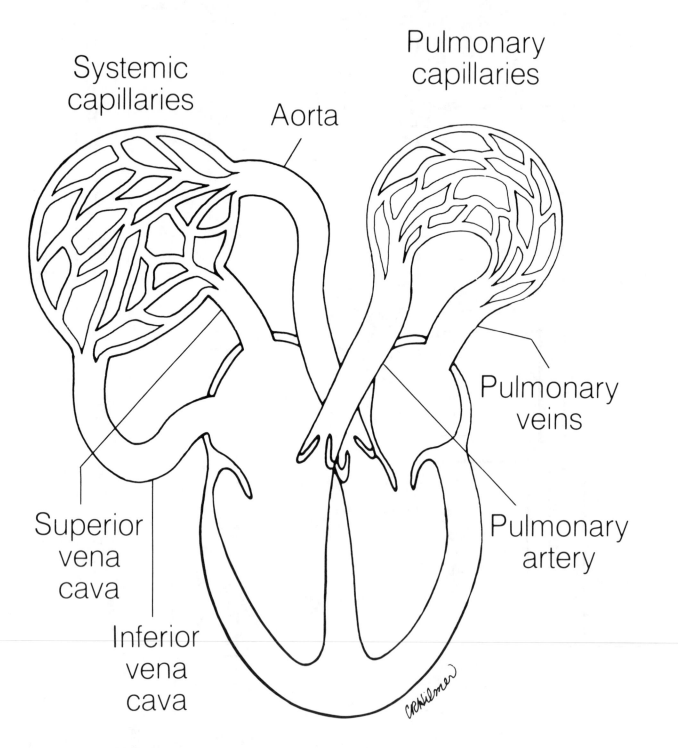

Systemic capillaries

Pulmonary capillaries

Aorta

Pulmonary veins

Superior vena cava

Pulmonary artery

Inferior vena cava

FIG. 19–1. *Systemic and pulmonary circulations. The right side of the heart pumps blood to the lungs, and the left side of the heart pumps blood to the systemic circulation*
Porth: Pathophysiology, 4th Edition
Copyright © 1994, J.B. Lippincott Company

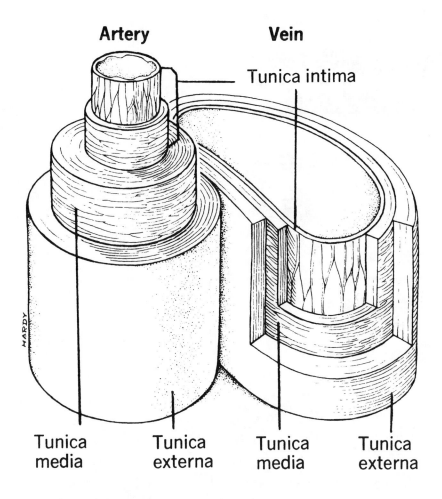

Artery   **Vein**

Tunica intima

Tunica
media

Tunica
externa

Tunica
media

Tunica
externa

FIG. 19–7. Medium-sized artery and vein showing the relative thickness of the three layers
Porth: Pathophysiology, 4th Edition
Copyright © 1994, J.B. Lippincott Company

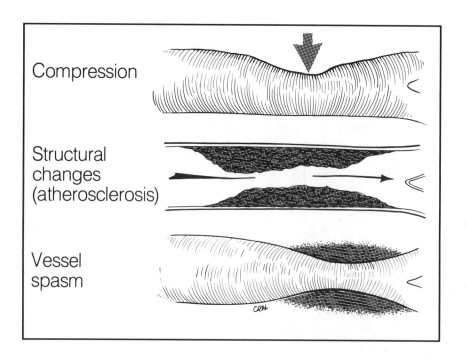

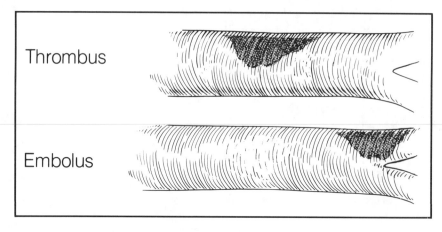

FIG. 20-1. Mechanisms of blood vessel occlusion
Porth: Pathophysiology, 4th Edition
Copyright © 1994, J.B. Lippincott Company

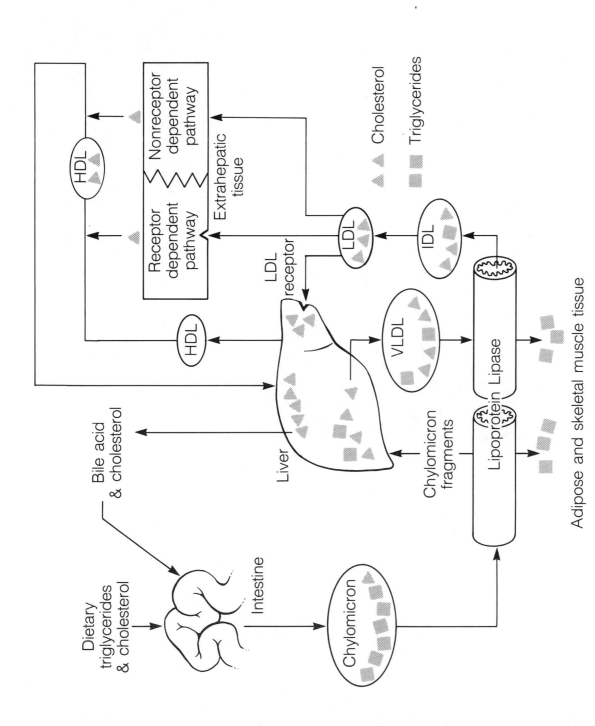

FIG. 20–4. Schematic representation of the exogenous and endogenous lipoprotein triglyceride and cholesterol transport
Porth: Pathophysiology. 4th Edition
Copyright © 1994, J.B. Lippincott Company

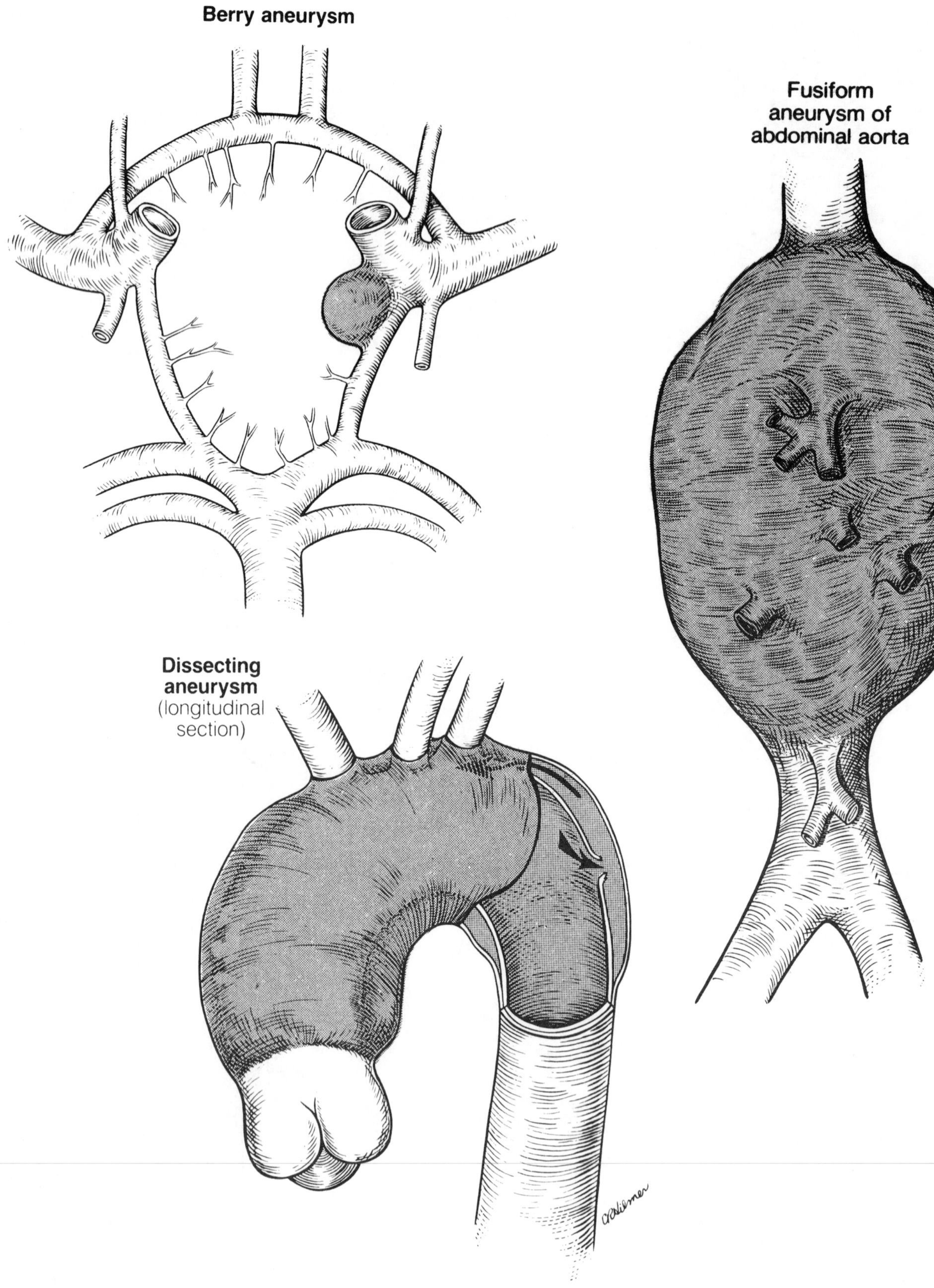

FIG. 20–5. Three forms of aneurysms—berry aneurysm in the circle of Willis, fusiform-type aneurysm of the abdominal aorta, and a dissecting aortic aneurysm
Porth: Pathophysiology, 4th Edition
Copyright © 1994, J.B. Lippincott Company

Systole

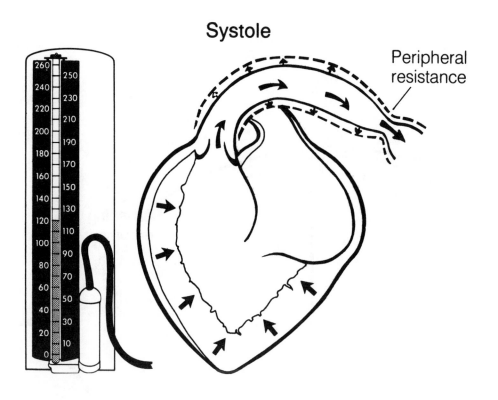

Peripheral resistance

Diastole

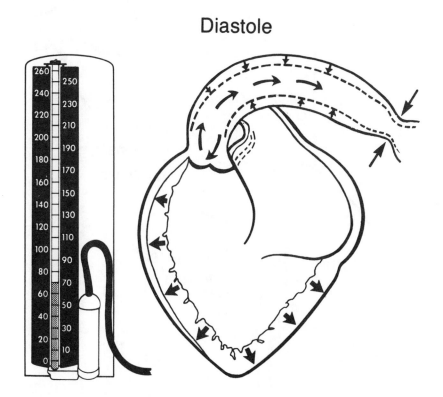

FIG. 21–2. Diagram of the left side of the heart. Systolic blood pressure (top). Diastolic blood pressure (bottom)
Porth: Pathophysiology, 4th Edition
Copyright © 1994, J.B. Lippincott Company

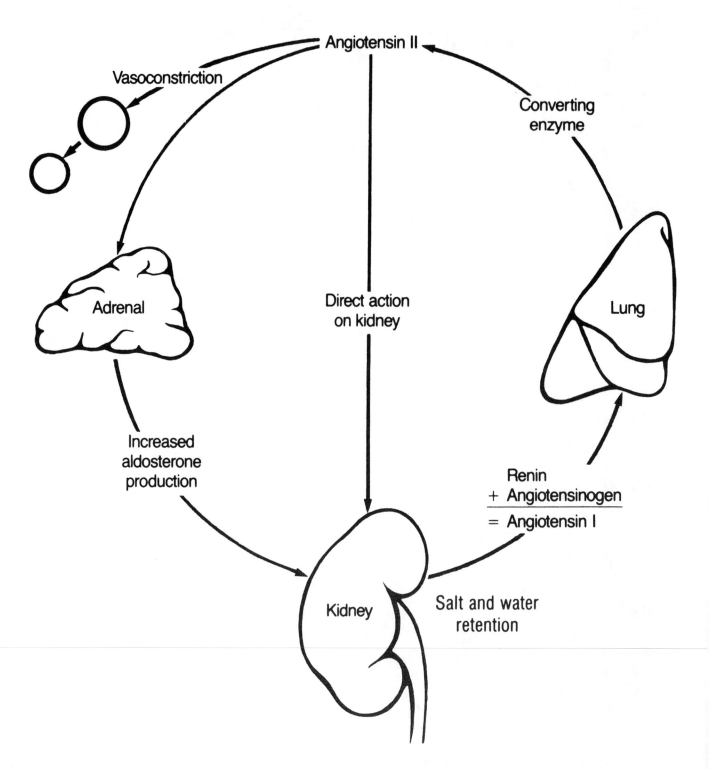

FIG. 21–4. Control of blood pressure by the renin-angiotensin-aldosterone system
Porth: Pathophysiology, 4th Edition
Copyright © 1994, J.B. Lippincott Company

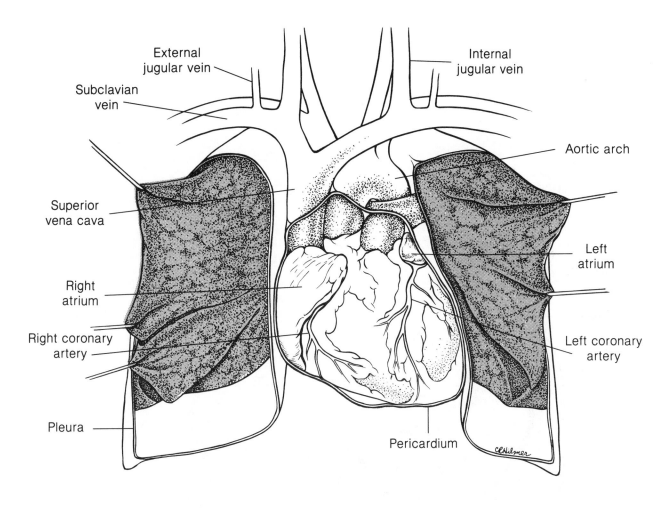

External
jugular vein

Internal
jugular vein

Subclavian
vein

Aortic arch

Superior
vena cava

Left
atrium

Right
atrium

Left coronary
artery

Right coronary
artery

Pleura

Pericardium

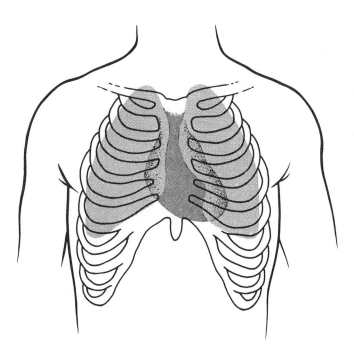

FIG. 22–1. (Top) Anterior view of the heart and great vessels (Bottom) Position of the
heart in relation to the skeletal structures of the chest cage
Porth: Pathophysiology, 4th Edition
Copyright © 1994, J.B. Lippincott Company

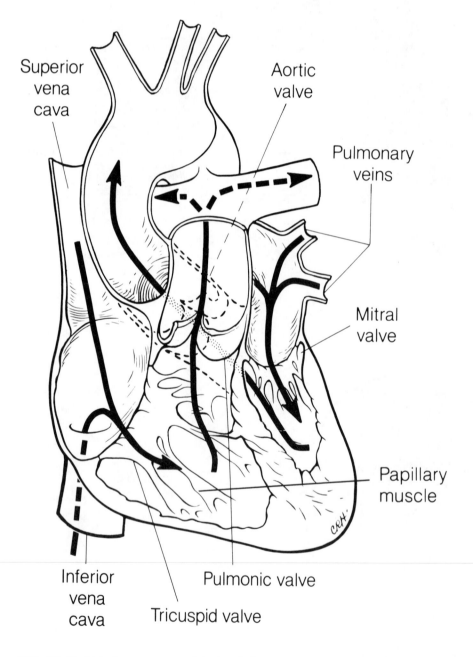

Superior vena cava

Aortic valve

Pulmonary veins

Mitral valve

Papillary muscle

Inferior vena cava

Pulmonic valve

Tricuspid valve

FIG. 22–5. Valvular structures of the heart. The atrioventricular valves are in an open position, and the semilunar valves are closed. There are no valves to control the flow of blood at the inflow channels (vena cava and pulmonary veins) to the heart

Porth: Pathophysiology, 4th Edition

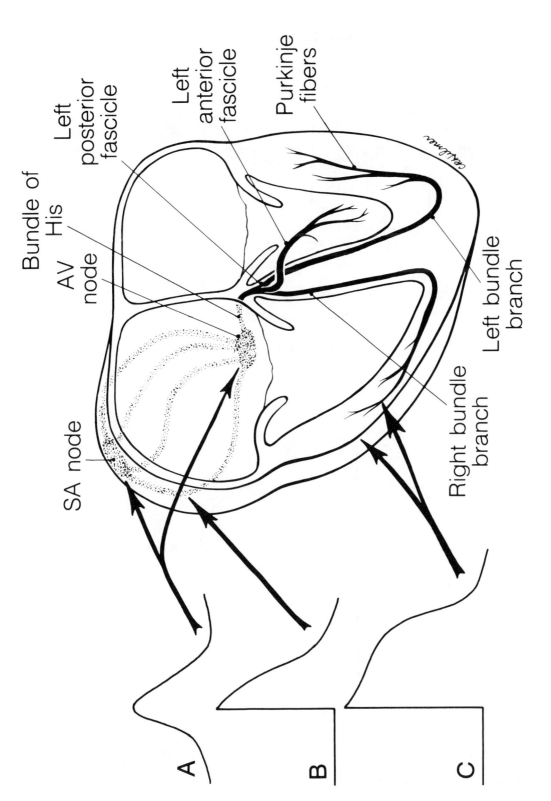

FIG. 22–7. Conduction system of the heart and action potentials (A) Action potential of SA and AV nodes; (B) atrial muscle action potential; (C) action potential of ventricular muscle and Purkinje fibers

Porth: Pathophysiology, 4th Edition
Copyright © 1994, J.B. Lippincott Company

Bundle of
Left
His
posterior
fascicle
Left
anterior
fascicle
Purkinje
fibers
AV
node
SA node
Right bundle
branch
Left bundle
branch

A

B

C

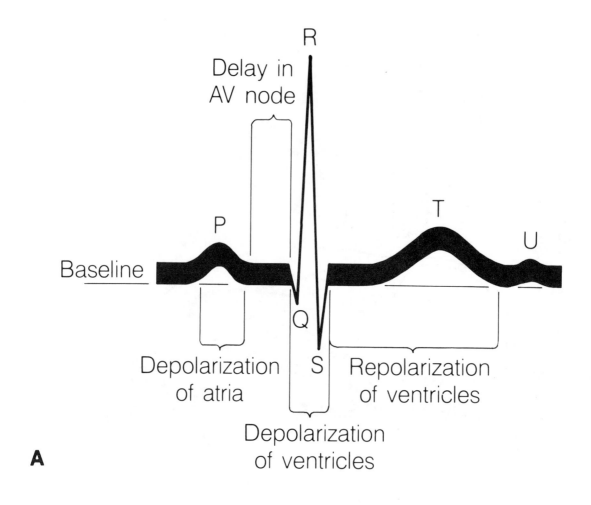

Delay in
AV node

R

P

Baseline

T

U

Q

S

Depolarization
of atria

Depolarization
of ventricles

Repolarization
of ventricles

A

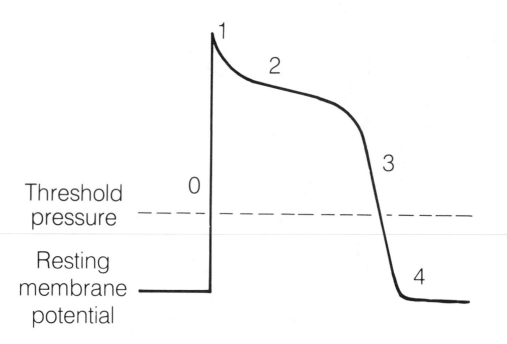

1

2

3

0

4

Threshold
pressure

Resting
membrane
potential

B

FIG. 22–9. Relation between electrocardiogram (A) and ventricular action potential (B)
Porth: Pathophysiology, 4th Edition
Copyright © 1994, J.B. Lippincott Company

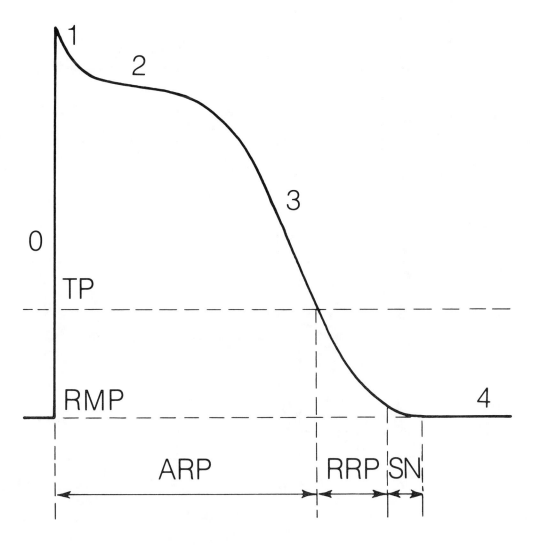

FIG. 22–11. Diagram of action potential of a ventricular muscle cell showing the RMP (resting membrane potential), ARP (absolute refractory period), RRP (relative refractory period), and SN (supernormal period)
Porth: Pathophysiology, 4th Edition
Copyright © 1994, J.B. Lippincott Company

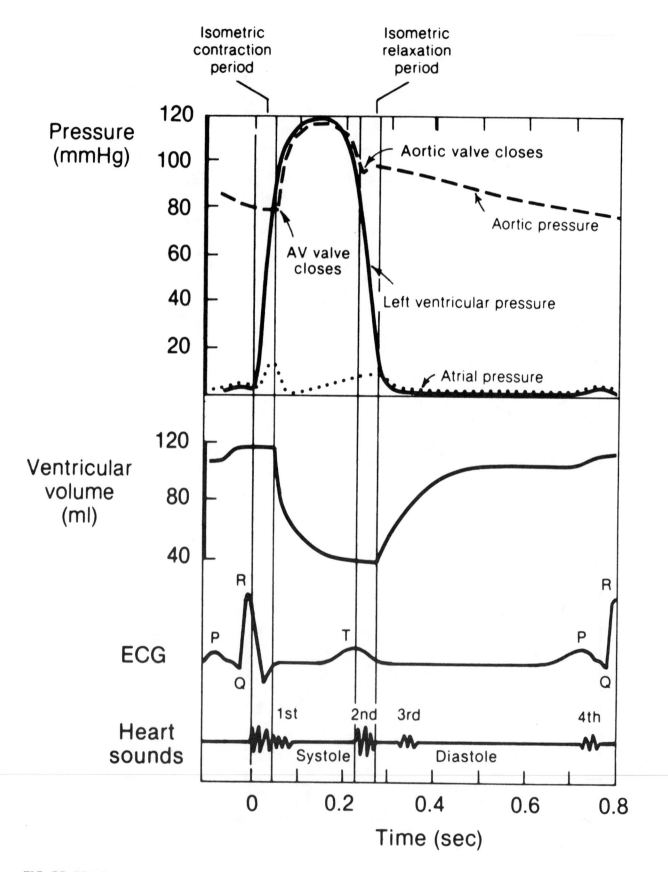

FIG. 22–12. Events in the cardiac cycle, showing changes in aortic pressure, left ventricular pressure, atrial pressure, left ventricular volume, the electrocardiogram, and heart sounds

Porth: Pathophysiology, 4th Edition

Copyright © 1994, J.B. Lippincott Company

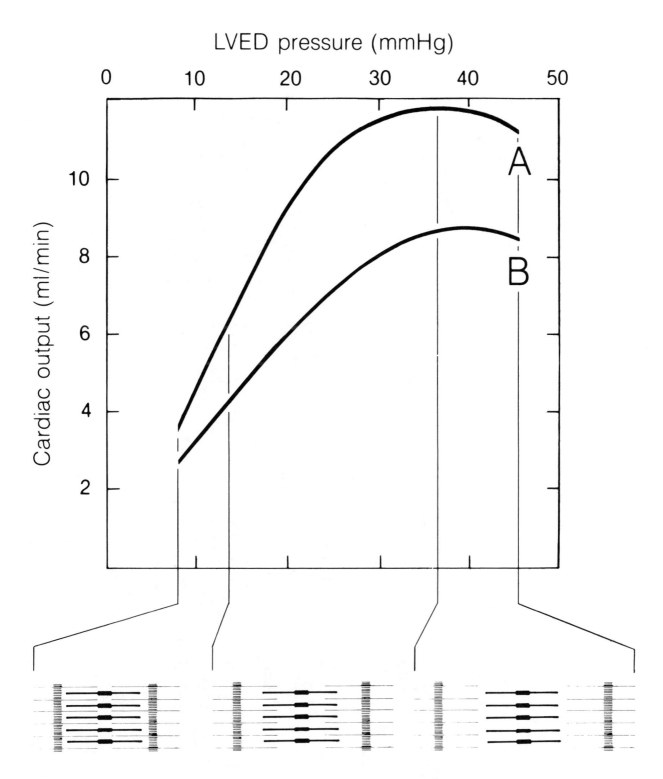

FIG. 22–13. (Top) Starling ventricular function curve. An increase in left ventricular end-diastolic (LVED) pressure produces an increase in cardiac output (curve A) by means of the Frank-Starling mechanism. In curve B, an increase in cardiac contractility produces an increase in cardiac output without a change in LVED volume and pressure (Bottom) Stretching of the actin and myosin filaments at the different LVED filling pressures

Porth: Pathophysiology, 4th Edition

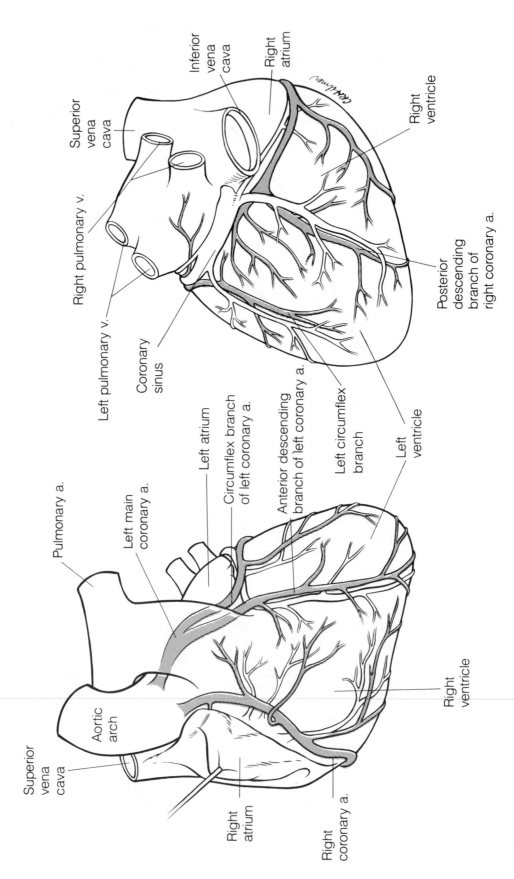

FIG. 23–2. Coronary arteries and some of the coronary sinus veins

Porth: Pathophysiology, 4th Edition

Copyright © 1994, J.B. Lippincott Company

Superior vena cava

Right pulmonary v.

Left pulmonary v.

Coronary sinus

Inferior vena cava

Right atrium

Right ventricle

Posterior descending branch of right coronary a.

Pulmonary a.

Left main coronary a.

Left atrium

Circumflex branch of left coronary a.

Anterior descending branch of left coronary a.

Left circumflex branch

Left ventricle

Aortic arch

Superior vena cava

Right atrium

Right coronary a.

Right ventricle

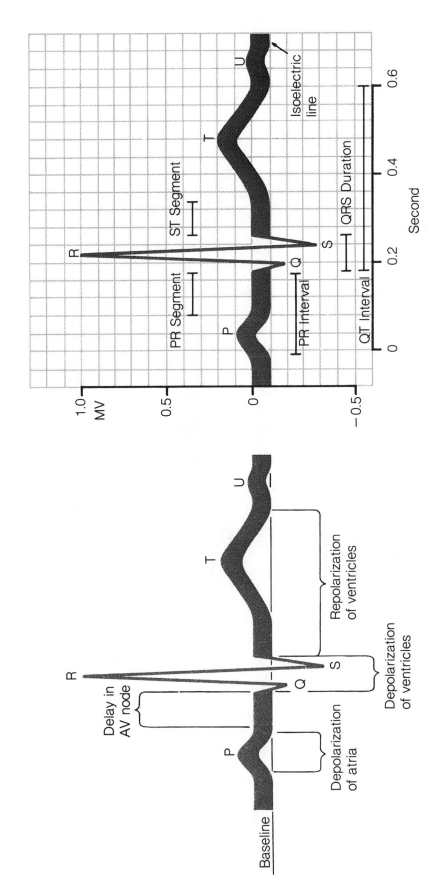

FIG. 23–11. Diagram of the electrocardiogram (lead III) and representative depolarization and repolarization of the atria and ventricle. The P wave represents atrial depolarization, the QRS complex ventricular depolarization, and the T wave ventricular repolarization. Atrial repolarization occurs during ventricular depolarization and is hidden under the QRS complex

Porth: Pathophysiology, 4th Edition
Copyright © 1994, J.B. Lippincott Company

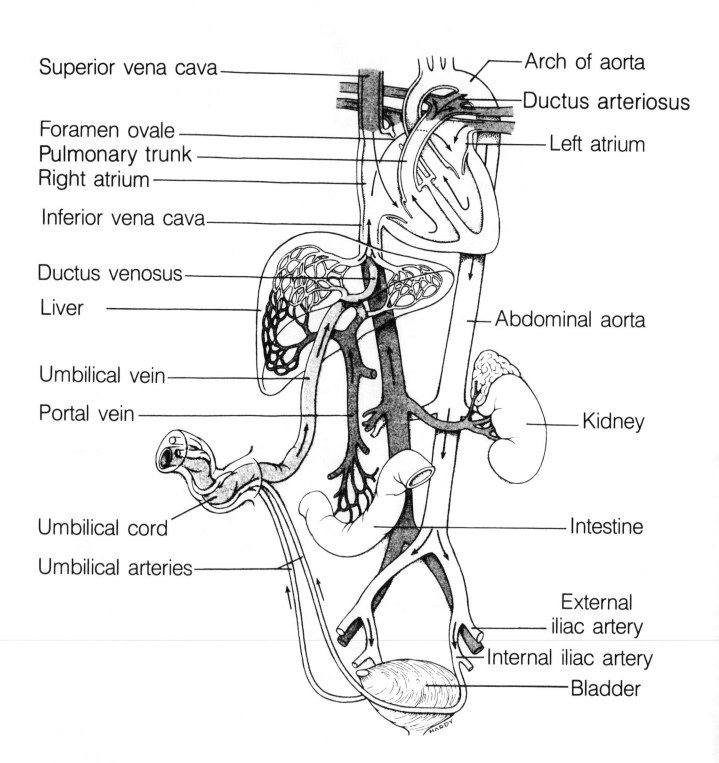

Superior vena cava

Foramen ovale
Pulmonary trunk
Right atrium

Inferior vena cava

Ductus venosus

Liver

Umbilical vein

Portal vein

Umbilical cord

Umbilical arteries

Arch of aorta

Ductus arteriosus

Left atrium

Abdominal aorta

Kidney

Intestine

External
iliac artery

Internal iliac artery

Bladder

FIG. 23–23. Fetal circulation
Porth: Pathophysiology, 4th Edition
Copyright © 1994, J.B. Lippincott Company

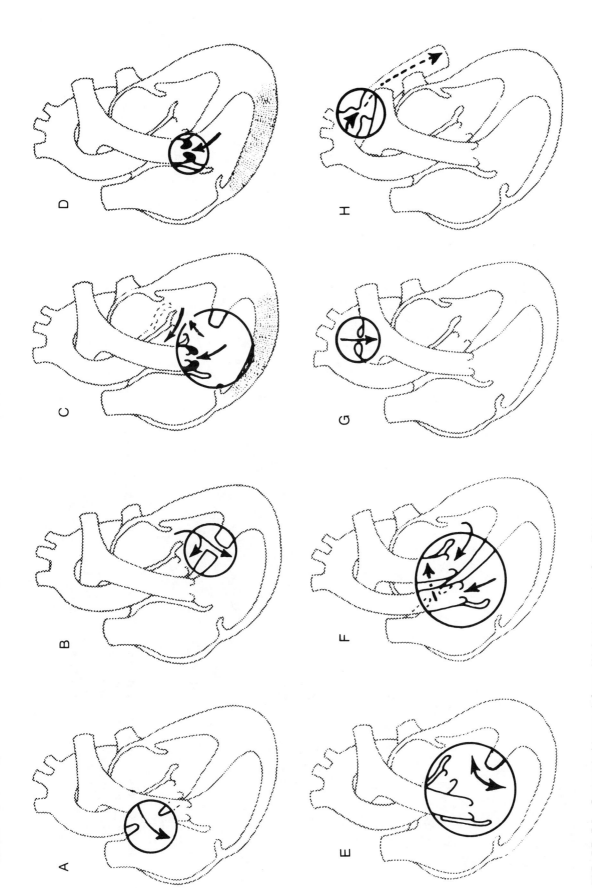

FIG. 23–24. Congenital heart defects. (A) Atrial septal defect. (B) Ventricular septal defect. (C) Tetralogy of Fallot. (D) Pulmonary stenosis, with decreased pulmonary blood flow and right ventricular hypertrophy. (E) Endocardial cushion defects. (F) Transposition of the great vessels. (G) Patent ductus arteriosus. (H) Postductal coarctation of the aorta

Porth: Pathophysiology, 4th Edition
Copyright © 1994, J.B. Lippincott Company

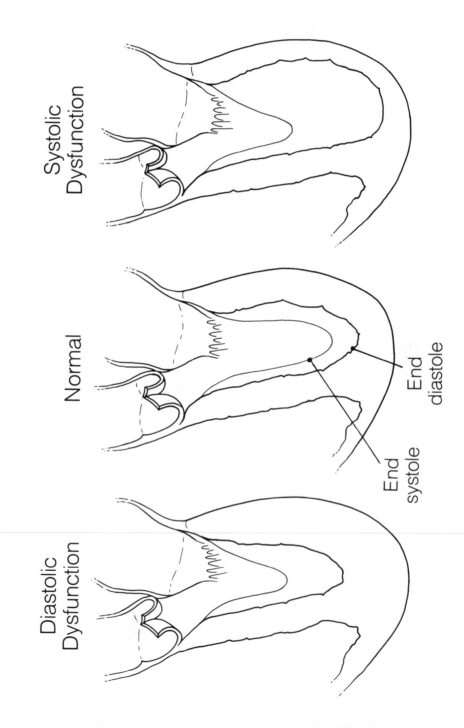

FIG. 24–3. Congestive heart failure due to systolic and diastolic dysfunction. Ejection fraction represents the difference between end diastolic function and end systolic volume. (Middle) Normal systolic and diastolic function with normal ejection fraction; (left) diastolic dysfunction with decreased ejection fraction due to decreased diastolic filling; (right) systolic dysfunction with decreased ejection fraction due to impaired systolic function

Porth: Pathophysiology, 4th Edition
Copyright © 1994, J.B. Lippincott Company

Right Heart Failure

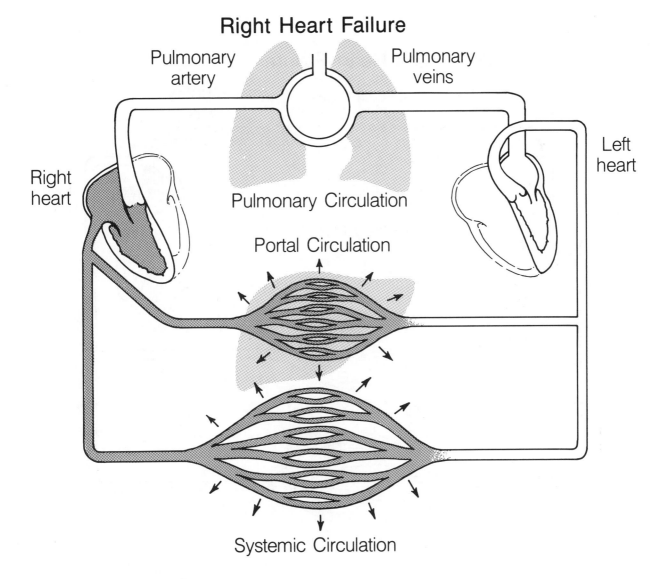

Pulmonary
artery

Pulmonary
veins

Right
heart

Left
heart

Pulmonary Circulation

Portal Circulation

Systemic Circulation

FIG. 24–4. Hemodynamic manifestations of right-sided heart failure
Porth: Pathophysiology, 4th Edition
Copyright © 1994, J.B. Lippincott Company

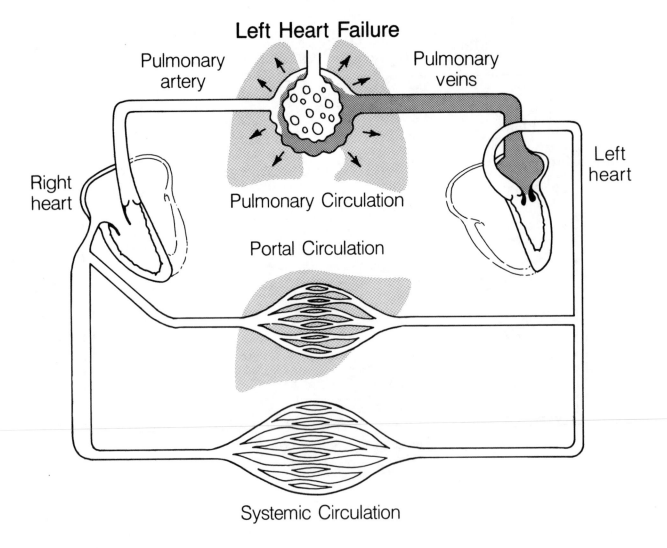

FIG. 24–5. Hemodynamic manifestations of left-sided heart failure
Porth: Pathophysiology, 4th Edition
Copyright © 1994, J.B. Lippincott Company

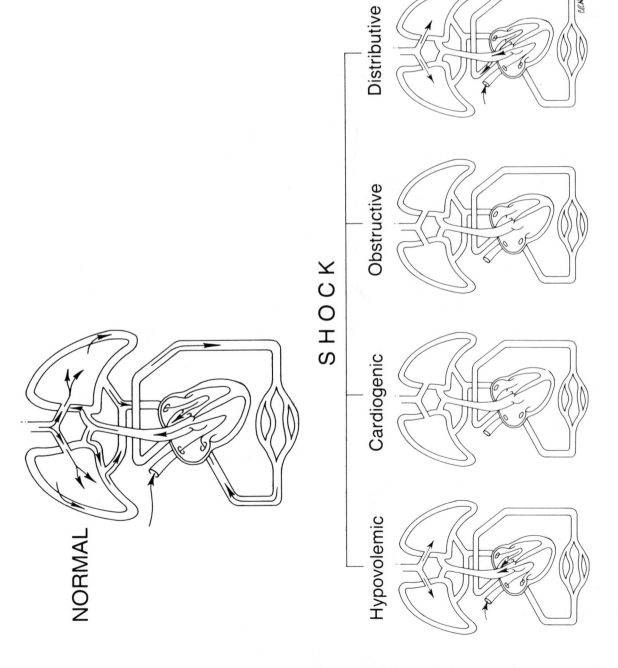

NORMAL

SHOCK

Hypovolemic   Cardiogenic   Obstructive   Distributive

FIG. 25-1. Types of Shock
Porth: Pathophysiology, 4th Edition
Copyright © 1994, J.B. Lippincott Company

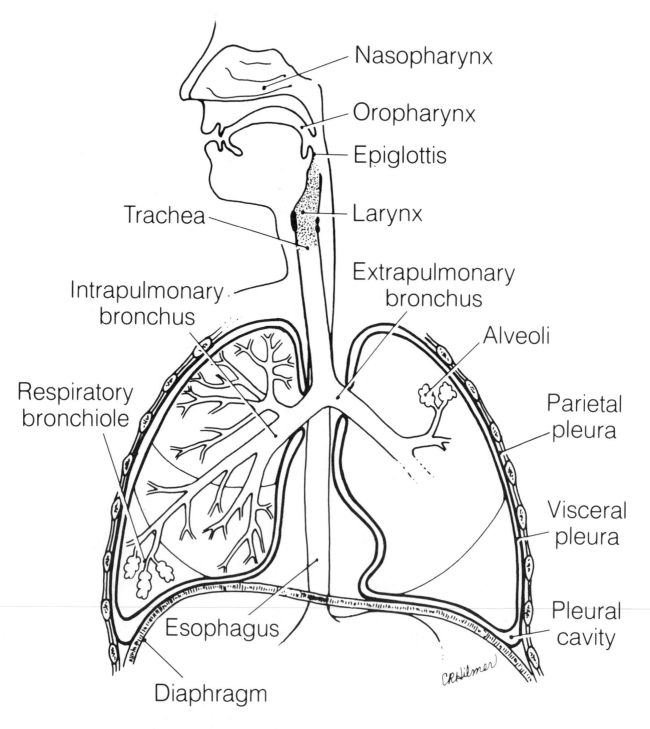

FIG. 26–1. Structures of the respiratory system
Porth: Pathophysiology, 4th Edition
Copyright © 1994, J.B. Lippincott Company

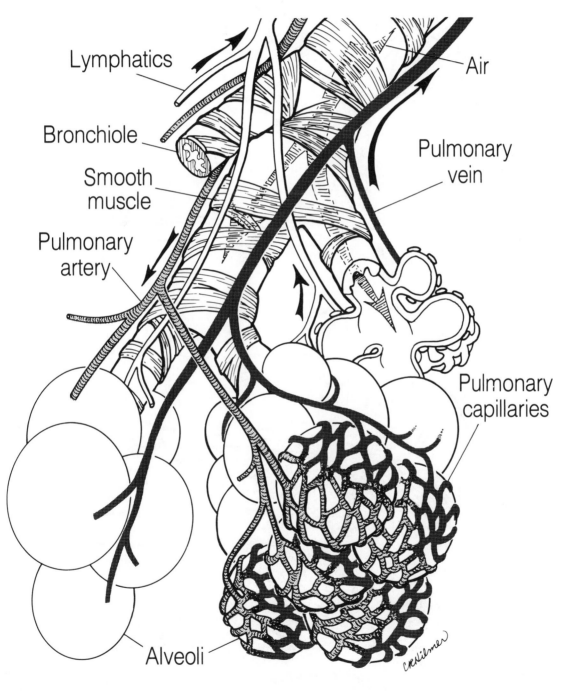

Lymphatics

Bronchiole

Smooth muscle

Pulmonary artery

Air

Pulmonary vein

Pulmonary capillaries

Alveoli

FIG. 26–5. Lobule of the lung showing the bronchial smooth muscle fibers, pulmonary blood vessels, and lymphatics
Porth: Pathophysiology, 4th Edition
Copyright © 1994, J.B. Lippincott Company

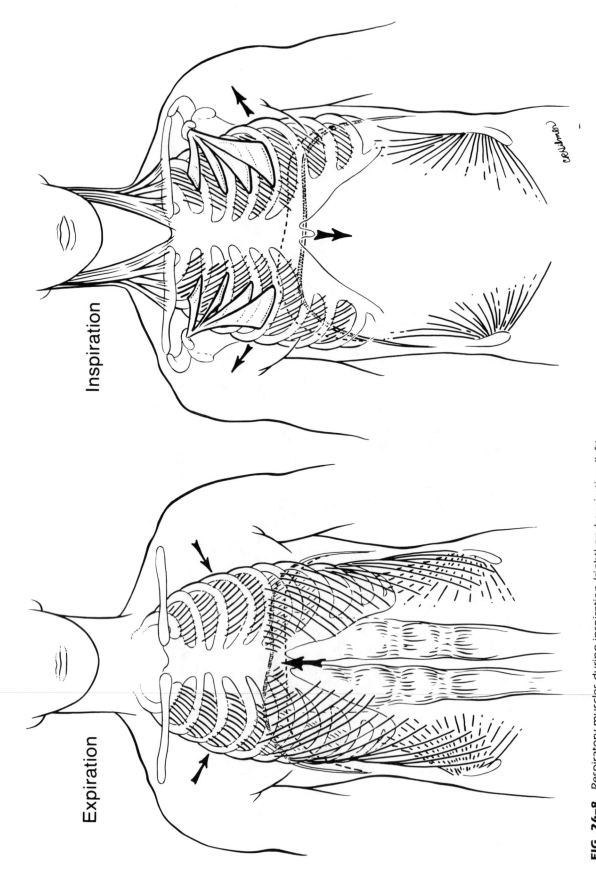

FIG. 26–8. Respiratory muscles during inspiration (right) and expiration (left)

Porth: *Pathophysiology, 4th Edition*

Copyright © 1994, J.B. Lippincott Company

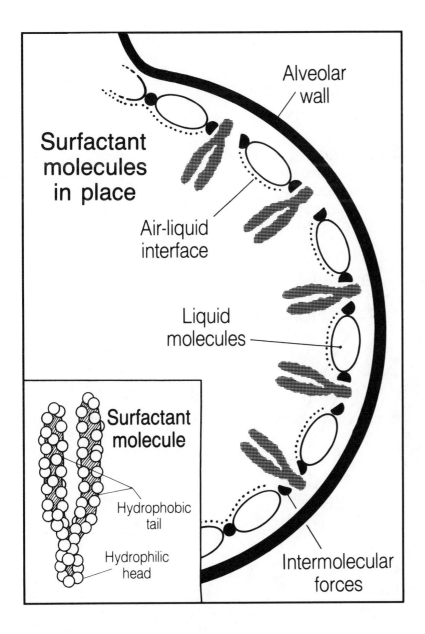

FIG. 26–11. *Alveolar wall depicting the surface tension resulting from the intermolecular forces at the air-liquid interface; the surfactant molecule with its hydrophobic tail and hydrophilic head; and its function in reducing surface tension by disrupting the intermolecular forces*
Porth: Pathophysiology, 4th Edition
Copyright © 1994, J.B. Lippincott Company

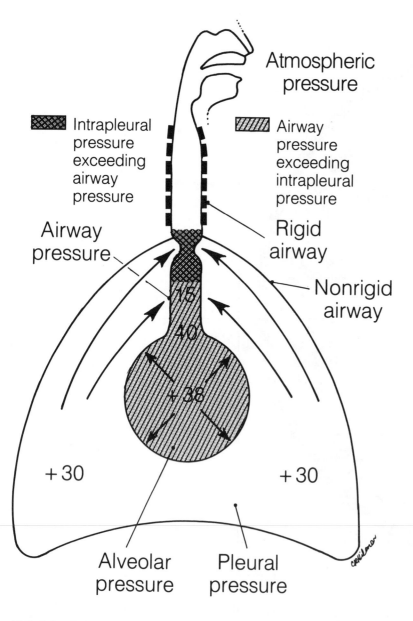

Atmospheric
pressure

Intrapleural
pressure
exceeding
airway
pressure

Airway
pressure
exceeding
intrapleural
pressure

Airway
pressure

Rigid
airway

Nonrigid
airway

15

40

+38

+30

+30

Alveolar
pressure

Pleural
pressure

FIG. 26–12. Mechanism that limits maximal expiratory flow rate. Forced expiration
increases intrapleural pressure, causing airway compression of nonrigid airways where
intrapleural pressure exceeds airway pressure
Porth: Pathophysiology, 4th Edition
Copyright © 1994, J.B. Lippincott Company

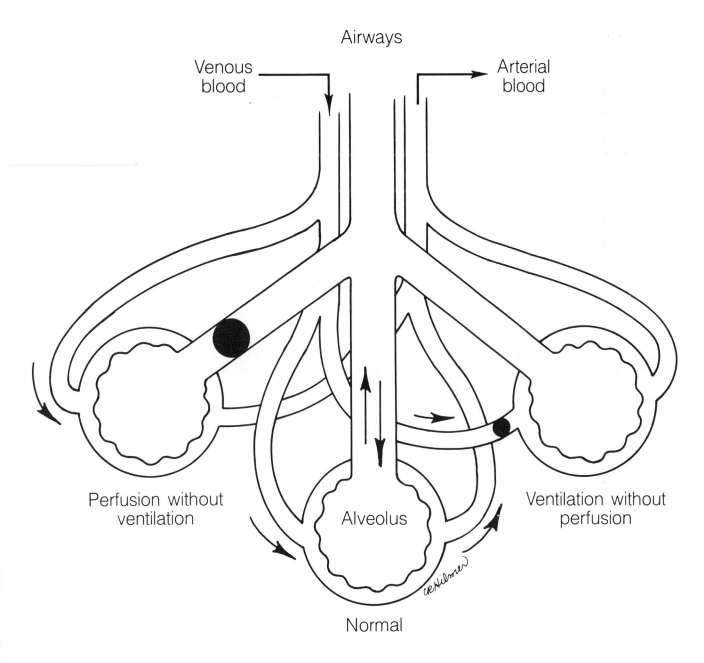

FIG. 26–14. Matching of ventilation and perfusion
Porth: Pathophysiology, 4th Edition
Copyright © 1994, J.B. Lippincott Company

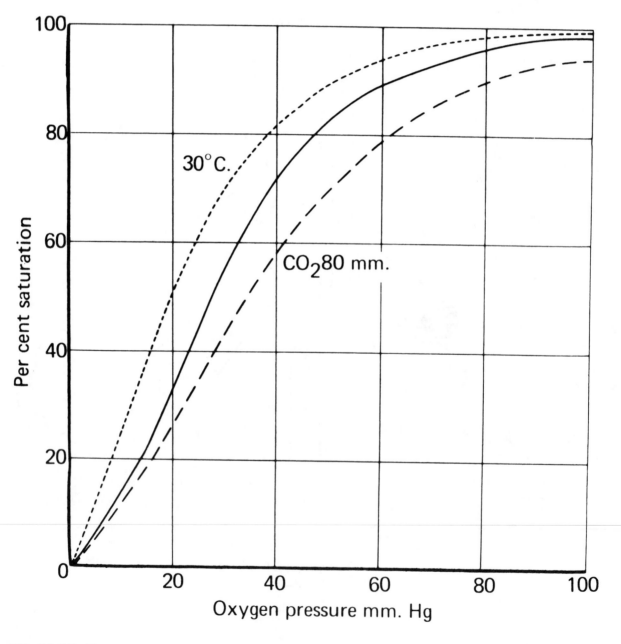

FIG. 26–15. The oxygen-hemoglobin dissociation curve
Porth: Pathophysiology, 4th Edition
Copyright © 1994, J.B. Lippincott Company

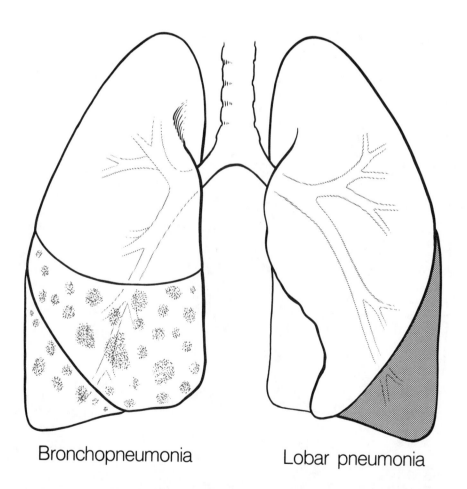

Bronchopneumonia   Lobar pneumonia

FIG. 27–1. Distribution of lung involvement in lobar and bronchial pneumonia

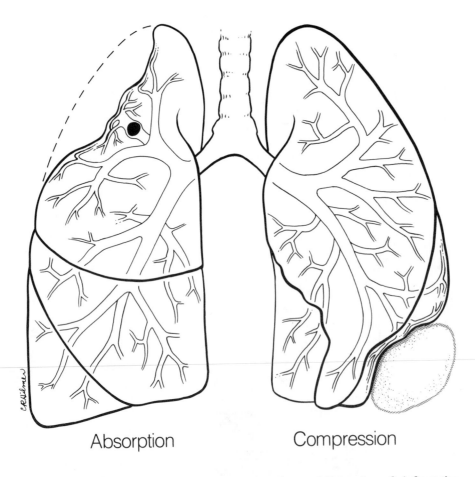

Absorption   Compression

FIG. 27–3. Atelectasis caused by airway obstruction and absorption of air from the involved lung area on the left and by compression of lung tissue on the right

Porth: Pathophysiology, 4th Edition

Copyright © 1994, J.B. Lippincott Company

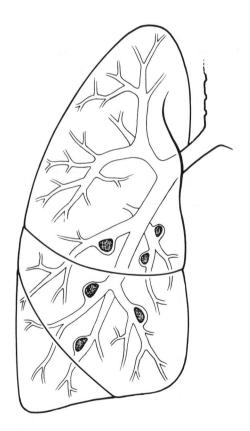

Bronchiectasis

FIG. 27–7. Bronchiectasis showing abnormal dilations of the large bronchi that are filled with inflammatory exudate

Porth: Pathophysiology, 4th Edition

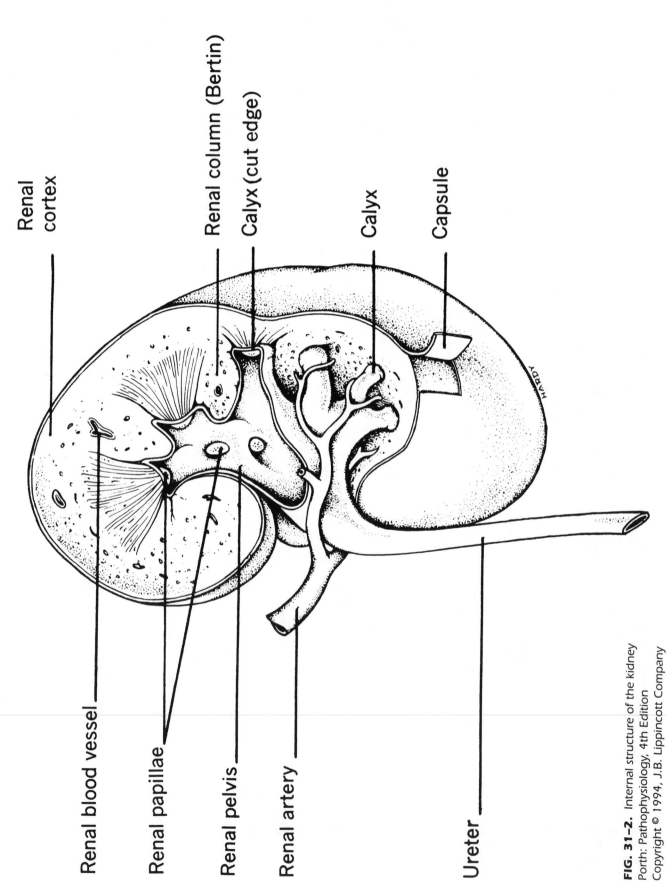

Renal cortex

Renal column (Bertin)

Calyx (cut edge)

Calyx

Capsule

Renal blood vessel

Renal papillae

Renal pelvis

Renal artery

Ureter

FIG. 31-2. Internal structure of the kidney
Porth: Pathophysiology, 4th Edition
Copyright © 1994, J.B. Lippincott Company

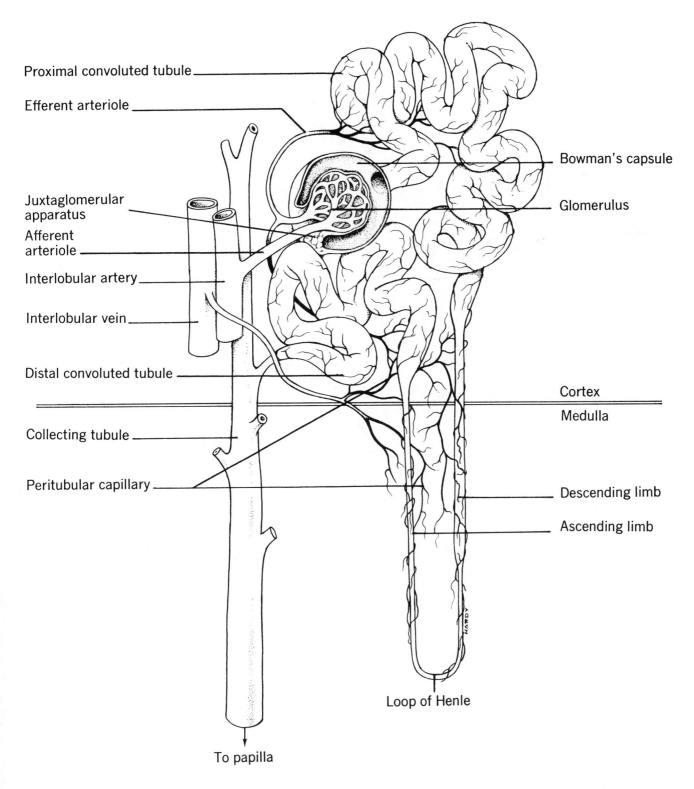

Proximal convoluted tubule

Efferent arteriole

Juxtaglomerular apparatus

Afferent arteriole

Interlobular artery

Interlobular vein

Distal convoluted tubule

Collecting tubule

Peritubular capillary

Bowman's capsule

Glomerulus

Cortex

Medulla

Descending limb

Ascending limb

Loop of Henle

To papilla

FIG. 31–3. Nephron, showing the glomerular and tubular structures along with the blood supply
Porth: Pathophysiology, 4th Edition
Copyright © 1994, J.B. Lippincott Company

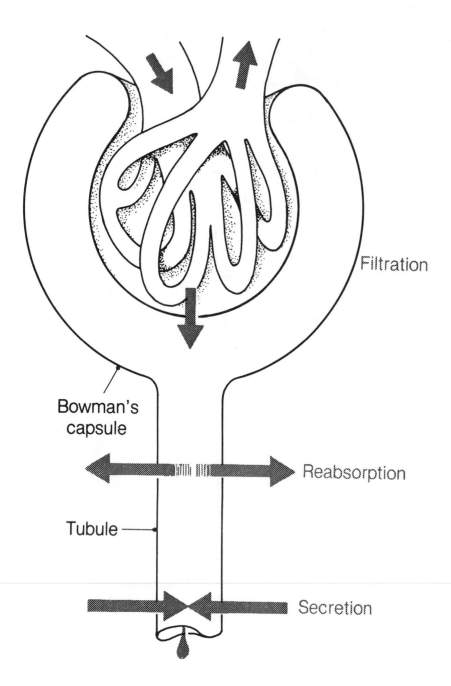

Filtration

Bowman's
capsule

Reabsorption

Tubule

Secretion

FIG. 31–7. Mechanisms of urine formation. The plasma is filtered in the glomerulus, and urine is formed as substances are reabsorbed or secreted into the filtrate
Porth: Pathophysiology, 4th Edition
Copyright © 1994, J.B. Lippincott Company

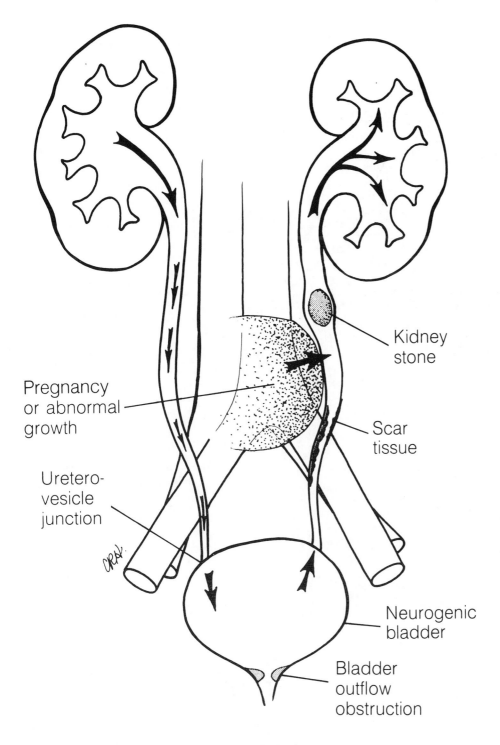

Kidney
stone

Pregnancy
or abnormal
growth

Scar
tissue

Uretero-
vesicle
junction

Neurogenic
bladder

Bladder
outflow
obstruction

FIG. 32–1. Locations and causes of urinary tract obstruction
Porth: Pathophysiology, 4th Edition
Copyright © 1994, J.B. Lippincott Company

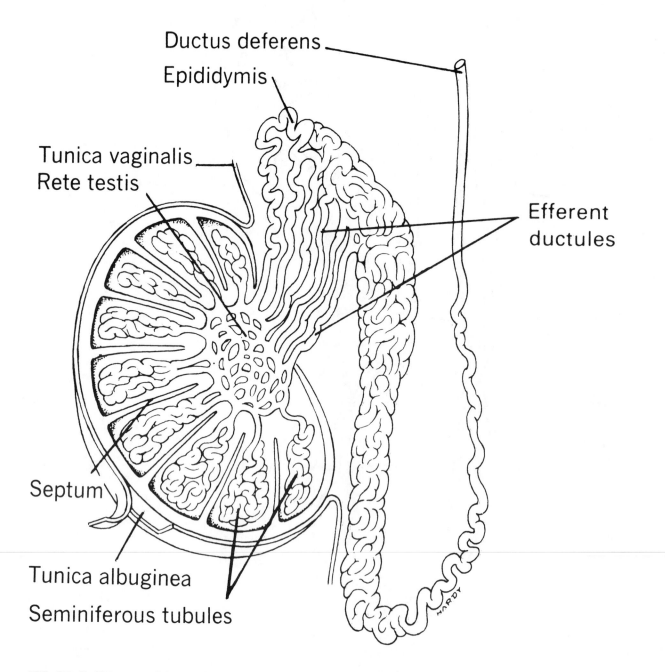

FIG. 35–2. The parts of the testes and epididymis
Porth: Pathophysiology, 4th Edition
Copyright © 1994, J.B. Lippincott Company

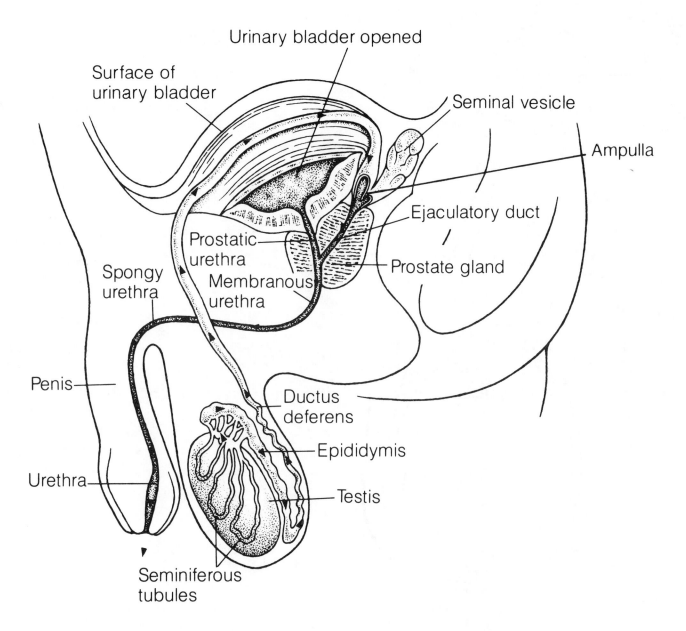

FIG. 35–3. The excretory ducts of the male reproductive system and the path that sperm follows as it leaves the testis and travels to the urethra

Porth: Pathophysiology, 4th Edition

Copyright © 1994, J.B. Lippincott Company

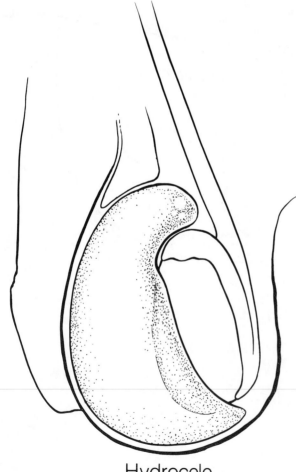

Hydrocele

FIG. 36–4. Hydrocele
Porth: Pathophysiology, 4th Edition
Copyright © 1994, J.B. Lippincott Company

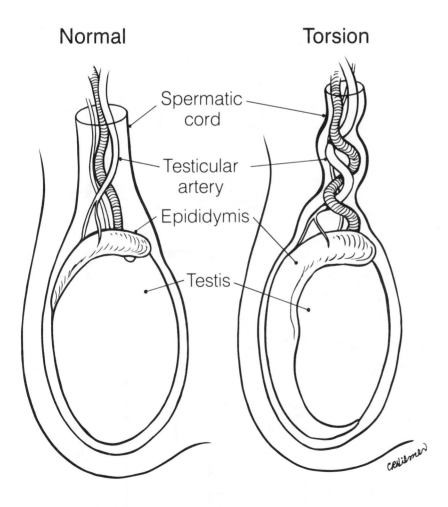

Normal   Torsion

Spermatic cord

Testicular artery

Epididymis

Testis

FIG. 36–5. Testicular torsion
Porth: Pathophysiology, 4th Edition
Copyright © 1994, J.B. Lippincott Company

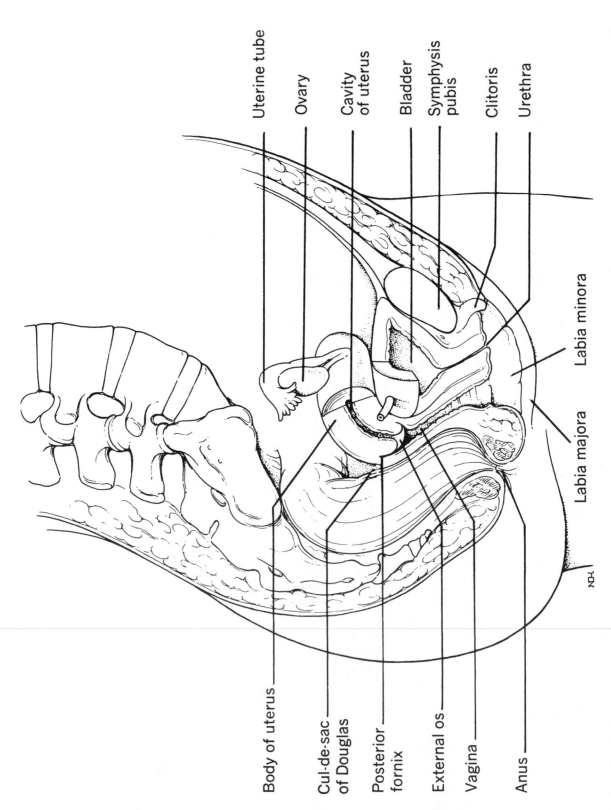

Uterine tube

Ovary

Cavity
of uterus

Bladder

Symphysis
pubis

Clitoris

Urethra

Labia minora

Labia majora

Body of uterus

Cul-de-sac
of Douglas

Posterior
fornix

External os

Vagina

Anus

FIG. 37-1. Female reproductive system as seen in sagittal section

Porth: Pathophysiology, 4th Edition

Copyright © 1994, J.B. Lippincott Company

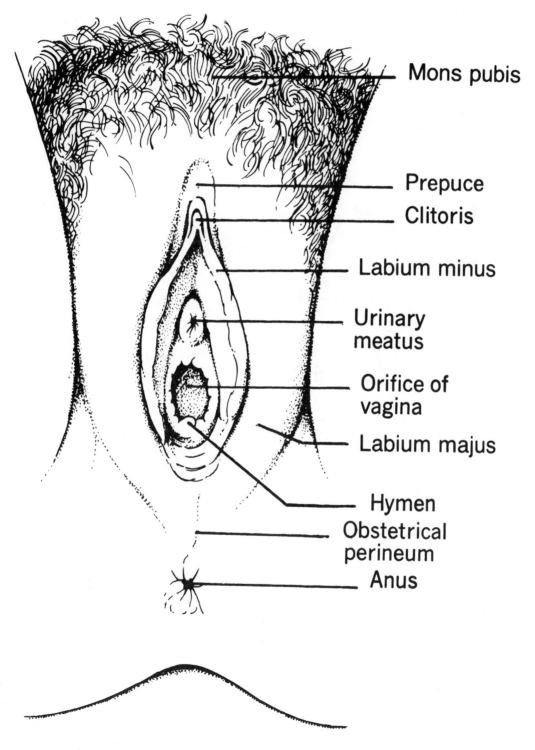

Mons pubis

Prepuce

Clitoris

Labium minus

Urinary
meatus

Orifice of
vagina

Labium majus

Hymen

Obstetrical
perineum

Anus

FIG. 37–2. External genitalia of the female
Porth: Pathophysiology, 4th Edition
Copyright © 1994, J.B. Lippincott Company

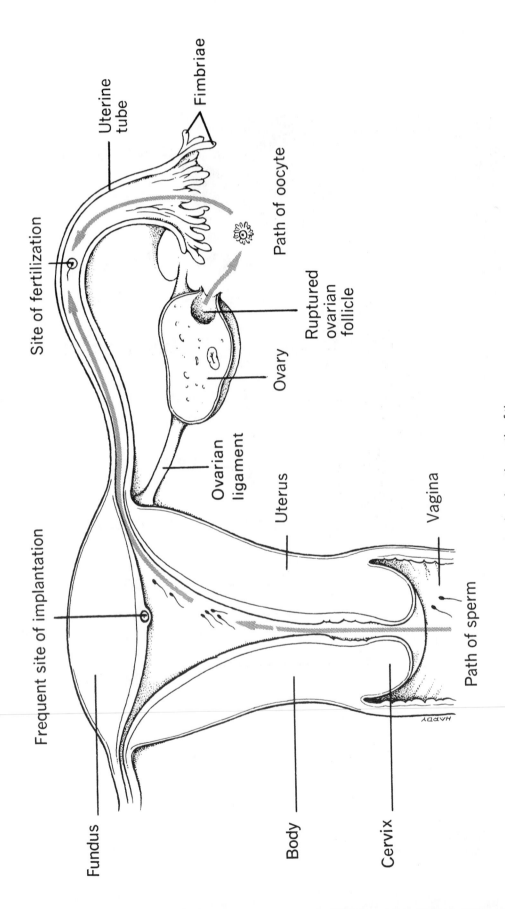

FIG. 37–3. Schematic drawing of female reproductive organs, showing the path of the oocyte as it moves from the ovary into the fallopian (uterine) tube; the path of sperm is also shown, as is the usual site of fertilization

Porth: Pathophysiology, 4th Edition

Copyright © 1994, J.B. Lippincott Company

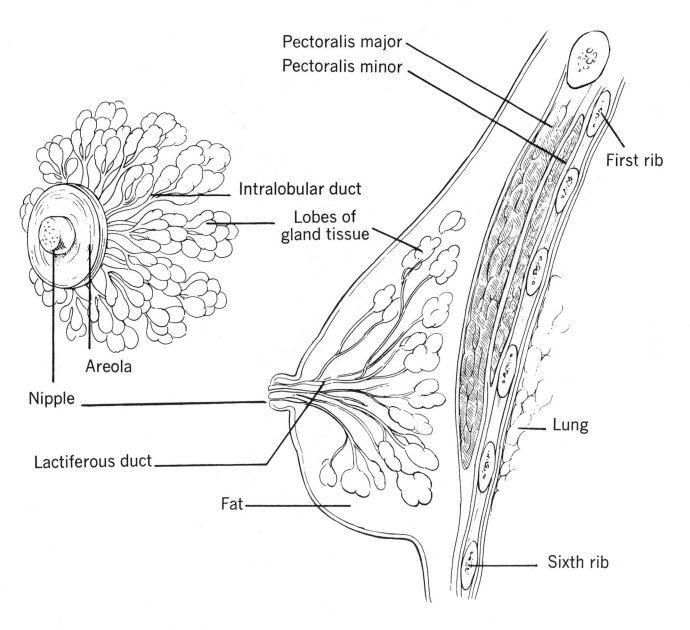

FIG. 37–8. The breast, showing the glandular tissue and ducts of the mammary glands
Porth: Pathophysiology, 4th Edition
Copyright © 1994, J.B. Lippincott Company

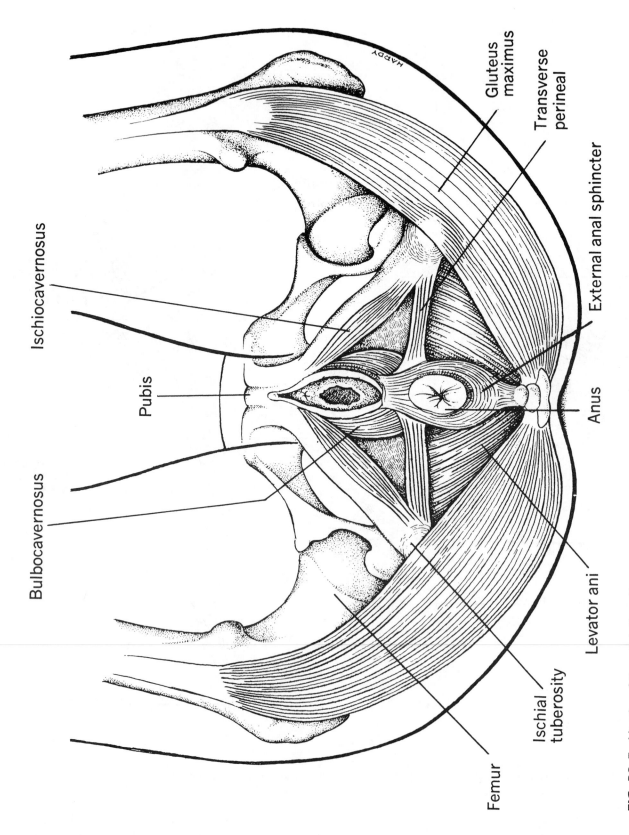

FIG. 38–5. Muscles of the pelvic floor (female perineum)
Porth: Pathophysiology. 4th Edition
Copyright © 1994, J.B. Lippincott Company

Ischiocavernosus

Bulbocavernosus

Pubis

Femur

Ischial tuberosity

Levator ani

Anus

External anal sphincter

Transverse perineal

Gluteus maximus

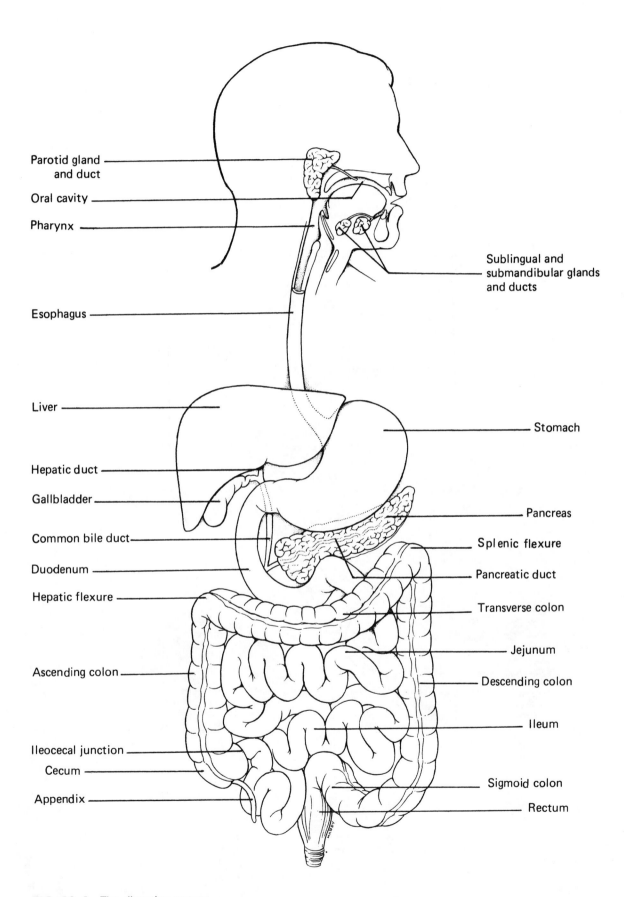

Parotid gland
and duct

Oral cavity

Pharynx

Sublingual and
submandibular glands
and ducts

Esophagus

Liver

Stomach

Hepatic duct

Gallbladder

Pancreas

Common bile duct

Splenic flexure

Duodenum

Pancreatic duct

Hepatic flexure

Transverse colon

Jejunum

Ascending colon

Descending colon

Ileum

Ileocecal junction

Cecum

Sigmoid colon

Appendix

Rectum

FIG. 40–1. The digestive system
Porth: Pathophysiology, 4th Edition
Copyright © 1994, J.B. Lippincott Company

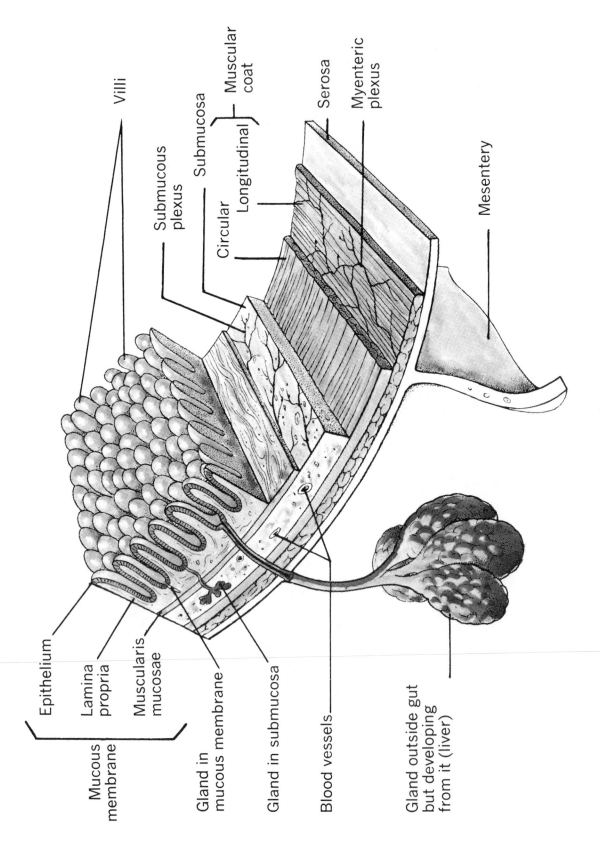

FIG. 40-6. Diagram of the four main layers of the wall of the digestive tube: mucosa, submucosa, muscular, and serosa (below the diaphragm)

Porth: Pathophysiology, 4th Edition

Copyright © 1994, J.B. Lippincott Company

Villi

Submucous plexus

Muscular coat

Submucosa

Circular

Longitudinal

Serosa

Myenteric plexus

Mesentery

Epithelium

Lamina propria

Muscularis mucosae

Mucous membrane

Gland in mucous membrane

Gland in submucosa

Blood vessels

Gland outside gut but developing from it (liver)

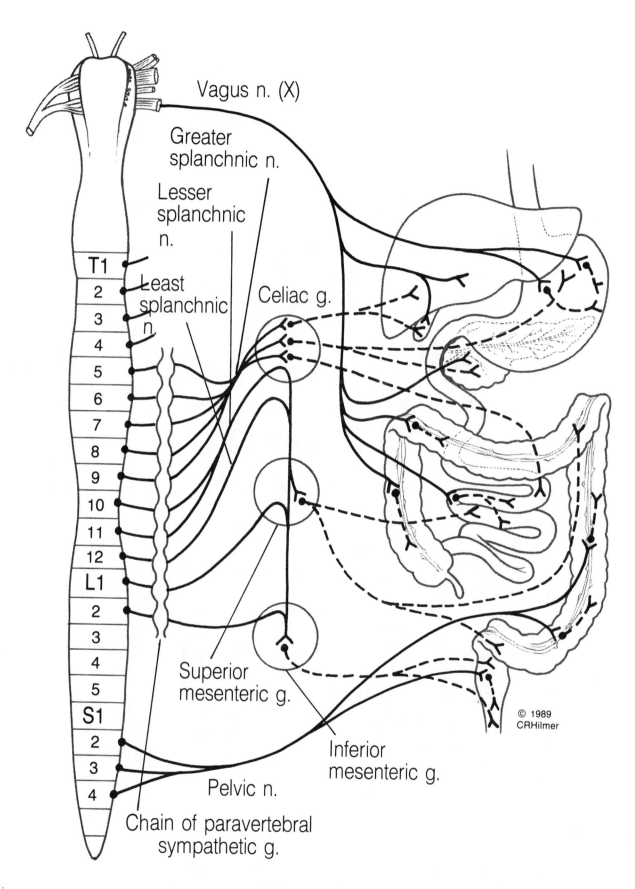

FIG. 40-7. The autonomic innervation of the gastrointestinal tract
Porth: Pathophysiology, 4th Edition
Copyright © 1994, J.B. Lippincott Company

Vagus n. (X)

Greater
splanchnic n.

Lesser
splanchnic
n.

Least
splanchnic
n.

Celiac g.

Superior
mesenteric g.

Inferior
mesenteric g.

Pelvic n.

Chain of paravertebral
sympathetic g.

© 1989
CRHilmer

T1
2
3
4
5
6
7
8
9
10
11
12
L1
2
3
4
5
S1
2
3
4

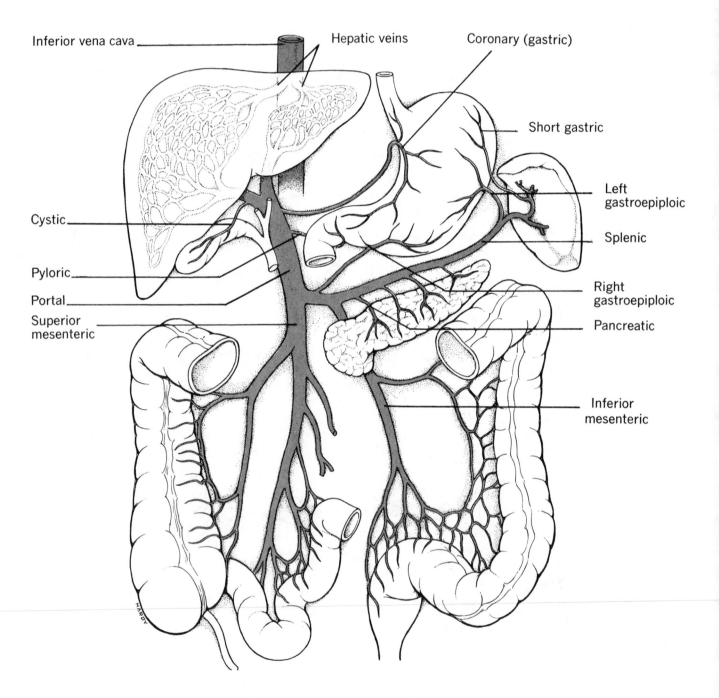

Inferior vena cava

Hepatic veins

Coronary (gastric)

Short gastric

Left gastroepiploic

Splenic

Cystic

Right gastroepiploic

Pyloric

Portal

Pancreatic

Superior mesenteric

Inferior mesenteric

FIG. 42–2. The portal circulation. Blood from the gastrointestinal tract, spleen, and pancreas travels to the liver by way of the portal vein before moving into the vena cava for return to the heart

Porth: Pathophysiology, 4th Edition

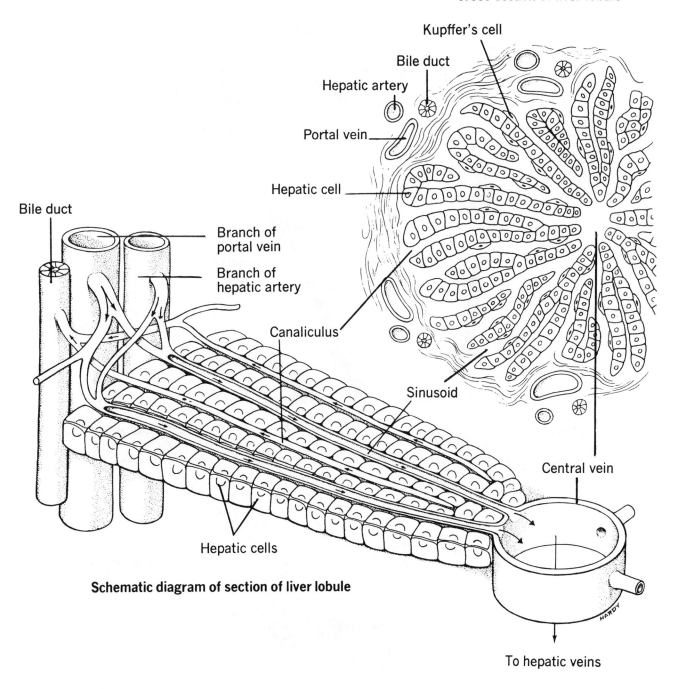

Cross section of liver lobule

Kupffer's cell

Bile duct

Hepatic artery

Portal vein

Hepatic cell

Canaliculus

Sinusoid

Central vein

Bile duct

Branch of portal vein

Branch of hepatic artery

Hepatic cells

Schematic diagram of section of liver lobule

To hepatic veins

Fig. 42–3. A section of liver lobule showing the location of the hepatic veins, hepatic cells, liver sinusoids, and branches of the portal vein and hepatic artery
Porth: Pathophysiology, 4th Edition
Copyright © 1994, J.B. Lippincott Company

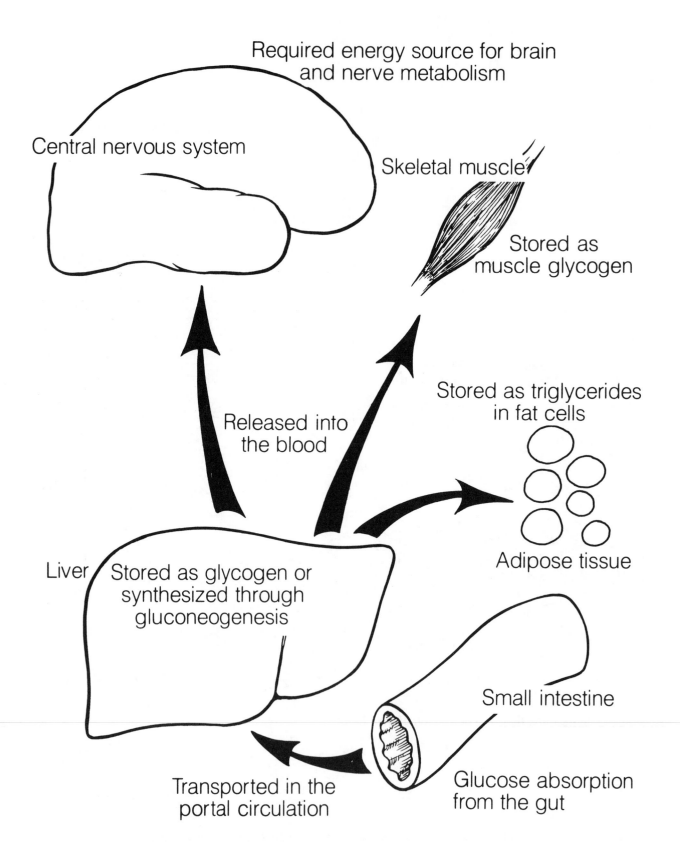

Required energy source for brain and nerve metabolism

Central nervous system

Skeletal muscle

Stored as muscle glycogen

Released into the blood

Stored as triglycerides in fat cells

Liver Stored as glycogen or synthesized through gluconeogenesis

Adipose tissue

Small intestine

Transported in the portal circulation

Glucose absorption from the gut

FIG. 43–2. Figure regulation of blood glucose by the liver
Porth: Pathophysiology, 4th Edition
Copyright © 1994, J.B. Lippincott Company

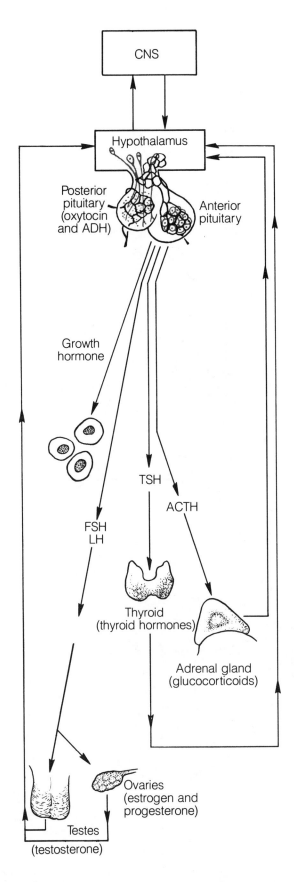

FIG. 44–4. Control of hormone production by hypothalamic-pituitary-target cell feedback mechanism. Hormone levels from the target glands regulate the release of hormones from the anterior pituitary by means of a negative feedback system
Porth: Pathophysiology, 4th Edition
Copyright © 1994, J.B. Lippincott Company

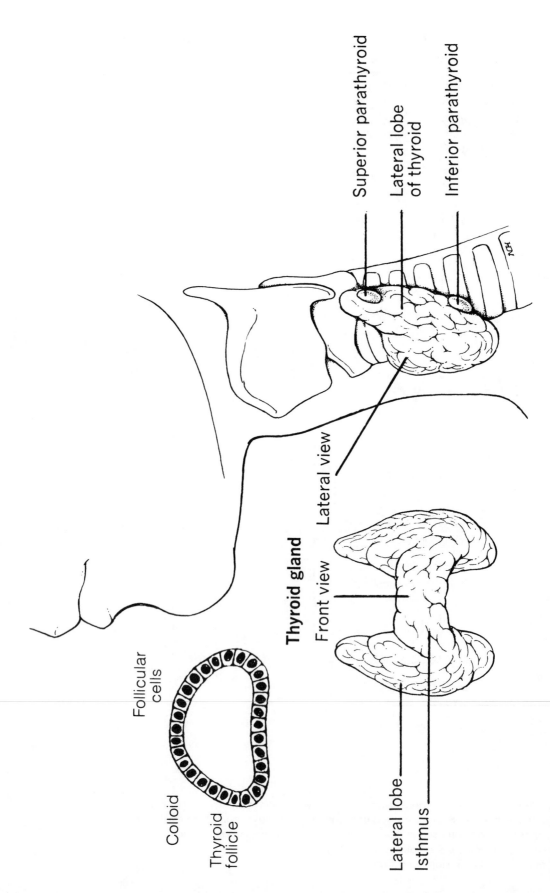

Follicular cells

Colloid

Thyroid follicle

Thyroid gland

Front view

Lateral view

Lateral lobe

Isthmus

Superior parathyroid

Lateral lobe of thyroid

Inferior parathyroid

FIG. 45–2. The thyroid gland and the follicular structure

Porth: Pathophysiology, 4th Edition

Copyright © 1994, J.B. Lippincott Company

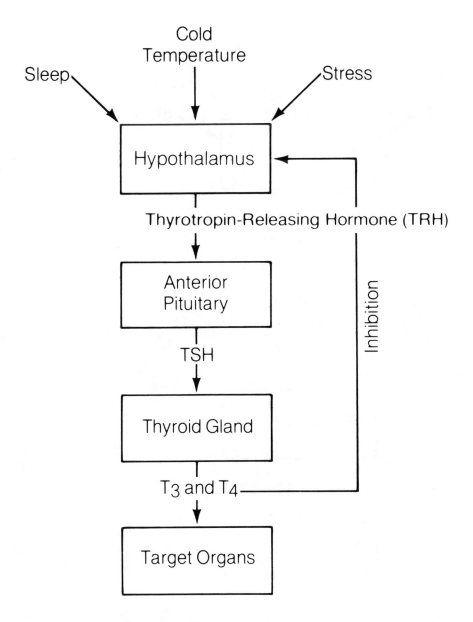

FIG. 45–4. The hypothalamic-pituitary-thyroid feedback system, which regulates the body levels of thyroid hormone
Porth: Pathophysiology, 4th Edition
Copyright © 1994, J.B. Lippincott Company

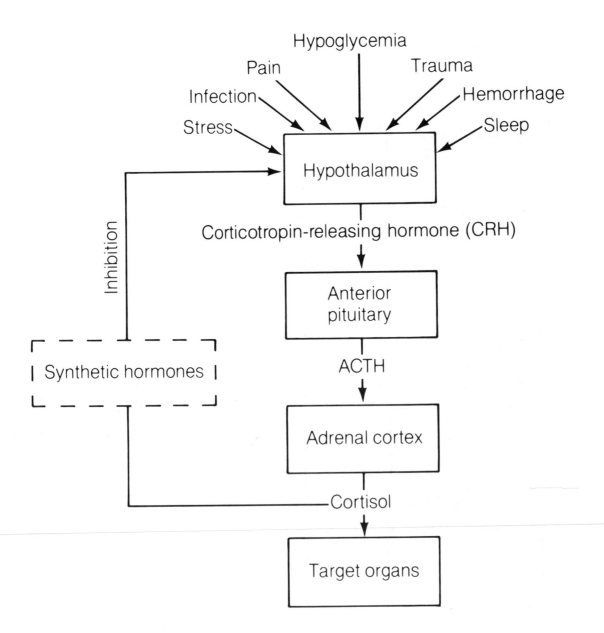

FIG. 45–9. The hypothalamic-pituitary-adrenal (HPA) feedback system that regulates glucocorticoid (cortisol) levels

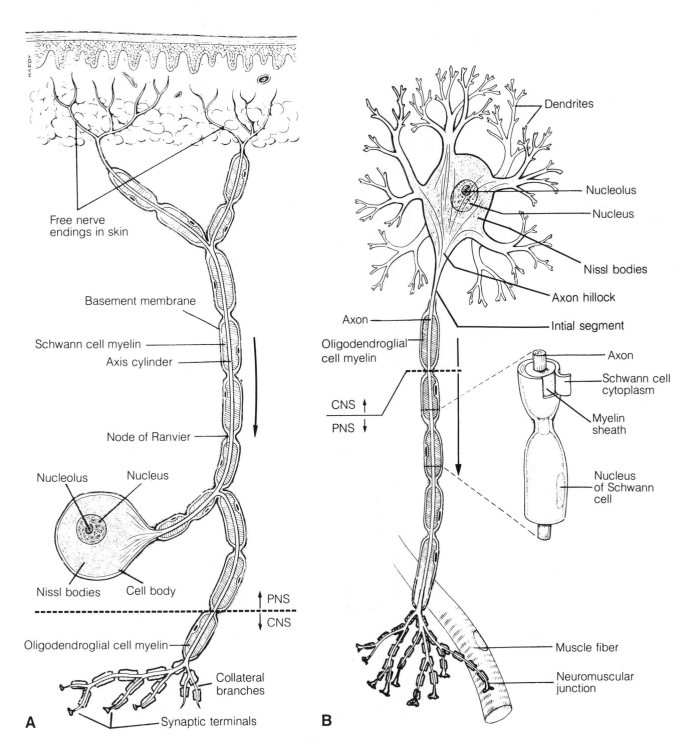

**Free nerve
endings in skin**

Basement membrane

Schwann cell myelin

Axis cylinder

Node of Ranvier

Nucleolus   **Nucleus**

Nissl bodies   **Cell body**

↑ **PNS**
↓ **CNS**

Oligodendroglial cell myelin

**Collateral
branches**

A   **Synaptic terminals**

Dendrites

Nucleolus

Nucleus

Nissl bodies

Axon hillock

Axon

Intial segment

**Oligodendroglial
cell myelin**

Axon

**Schwann cell
cytoplasm**

CNS ↑

PNS ↓

**Myelin
sheath**

**Nucleus
of Schwann
cell**

Muscle fiber

**Neuromuscular
junction**

B

FIG. 47–7. (A) A typical afferent neuron that carries information from surface receptors
(in this case, the skin) to the central nervous system (CNS) (B) Myelinated efferent neuron
with axon entering the peripheral nervous system (PNS) to innervate skeletal muscle cells
Porth: Pathophysiology, 4th Edition
Copyright © 1994, J.B. Lippincott Company

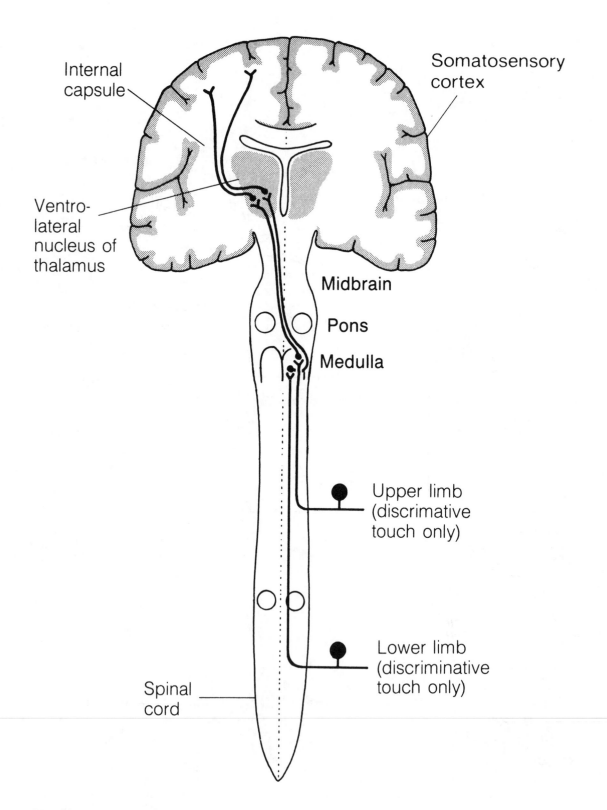

FIG. 48–3. Discriminative pathway. This pathway is an ascending system for rapid transmission of sensations that relate joint movement (kinesthesis), body position (proprioception), vibration, and delicate touch

Porth: Pathophysiology, 4th Edition

Copyright © 1994, J.B. Lippincott Company

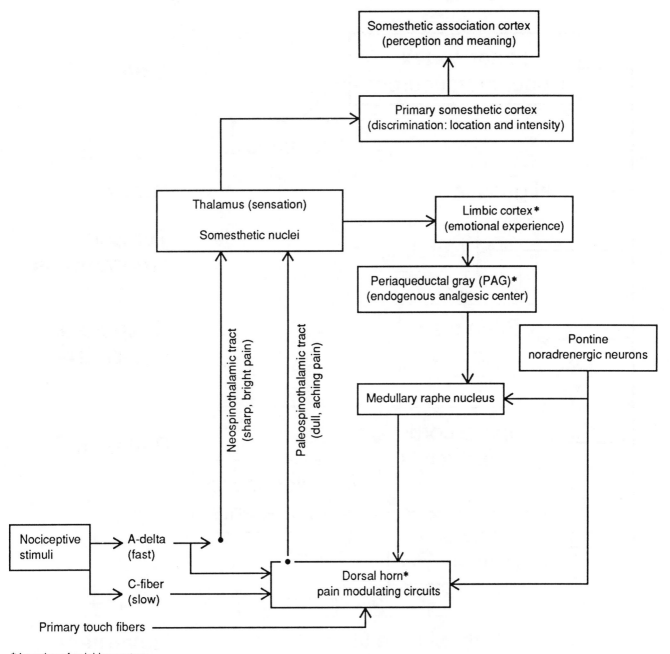

FIG. 48–7. Primary pain pathways
Porth: Pathophysiology, 4th Edition
Copyright © 1994, J.B. Lippincott Company

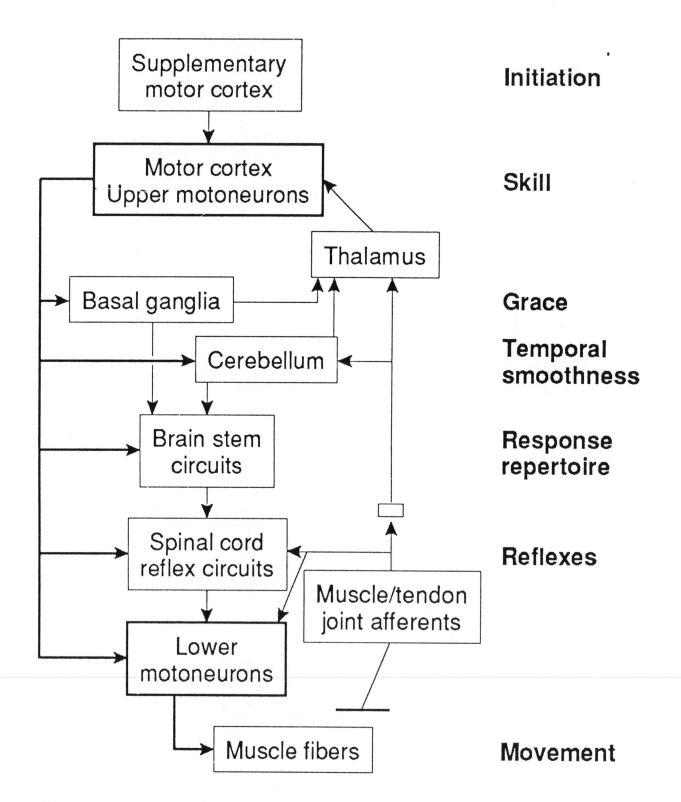

FIG. 50–1. Diagram of neural pathways for control of motor function
Porth: Pathophysiology, 4th Edition
Copyright © 1994, J.B. Lippincott Company

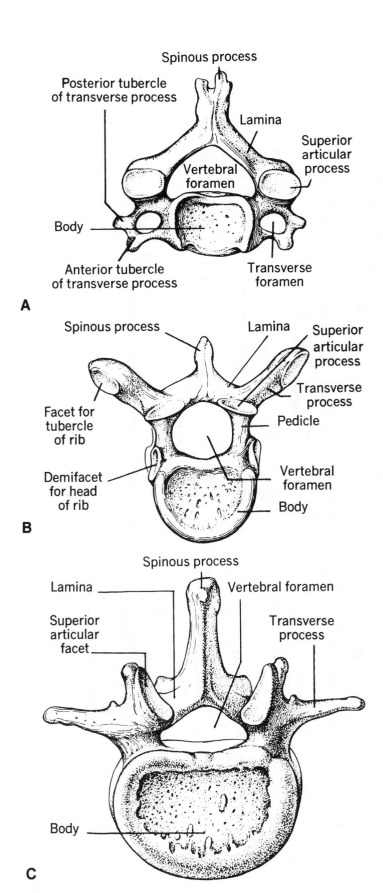

FIG. 50–13. Views of the three types of vertebrae. (A) Fourth cervical vertebra, superior aspect; (B) sixth thoracic vertebra, superior aspect; (C) third lumbar vertebra, superior aspect

Porth: Pathophysiology, 4th Edition

Copyright © 1994, J.B. Lippincott Company

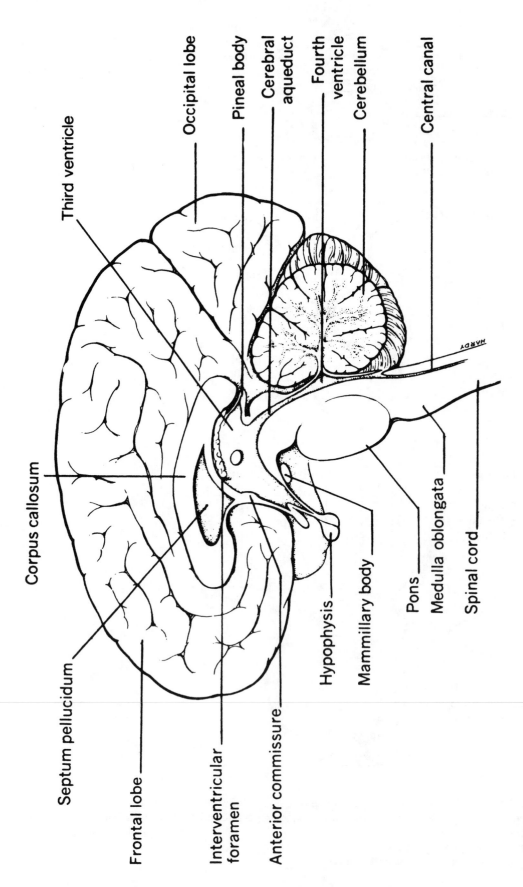

FIG. 51–3. Midsagittal section of the brain
Porth: Pathophysiology, 4th Edition
Copyright © 1994, J.B. Lippincott Company

Third ventricle

Occipital lobe

Pineal body

Cerebral aqueduct

Fourth ventricle

Cerebellum

Central canal

Corpus callosum

Septum pellucidum

Frontal lobe

Interventricular foramen

Anterior commissure

Hypophysis

Mammillary body

Pons

Medulla oblongata

Spinal cord

HARDY

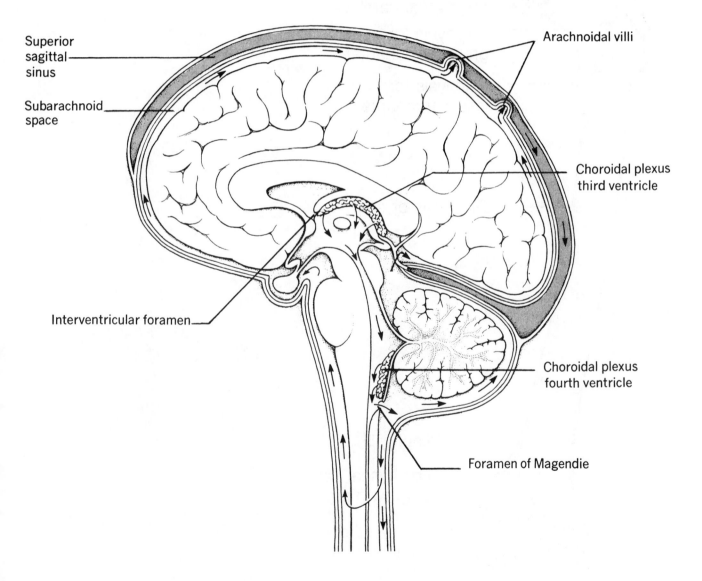

Superior sagittal sinus

Subarachnoid space

Arachnoidal villi

Choroidal plexus third ventricle

Interventricular foramen

Choroidal plexus fourth ventricle

Foramen of Magendie

FIG. 51–11. The flow of cerebrospinal fluid from the time of its formation from blood in the choroid plexuses until its return to the blood in the superior sagittal sinus. (Note: Plexuses in the lateral ventricles are not illustrated)
Porth: Pathophysiology, 4th Edition
Copyright © 1994, J.B. Lippincott Company

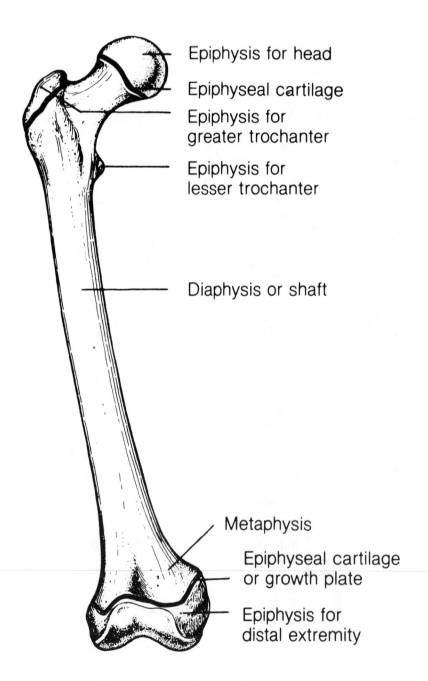

Epiphysis for head

Epiphyseal cartilage

Epiphysis for
greater trochanter

Epiphysis for
lesser trochanter

Diaphysis or shaft

Metaphysis

Epiphyseal cartilage
or growth plate

Epiphysis for
distal extremity

FIG. 55–3. A femur, showing epiphyseal cartilages for the head, metaphysis, trochanters, and distal end of the bone
Porth: Pathophysiology, 4th Edition
Copyright © 1994, J.B. Lippincott Company

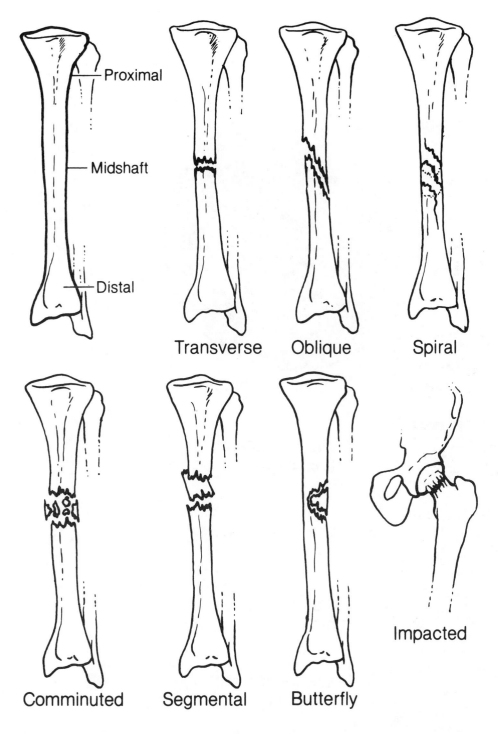

FIG. 56–2. Classification of fractures. Fractures are classified according to location (proximal, midshaft, or distal), the direction of fracture line (transverse, oblique, spiral), and type (comminuted, segmental, butterfly, or impacted)

Porth: Pathophysiology, 4th Edition

Copyright © 1994, J.B. Lippincott Company

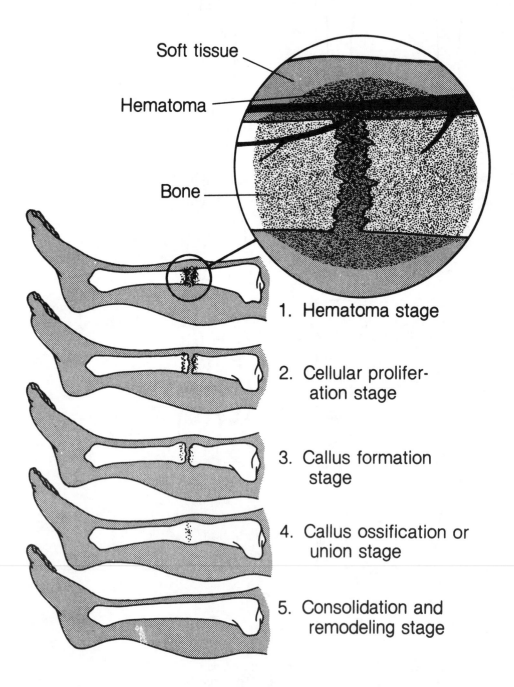

Soft tissue

Hematoma

Bone

1. Hematoma stage

2. Cellular prolifer-
   ation stage

3. Callus formation
   stage

4. Callus ossification or
   union stage

5. Consolidation and
   remodeling stage

FIG. 56–4. Healing of a fracture
Porth: Pathophysiology, 4th Edition
Copyright © 1994, J.B. Lippincott Company

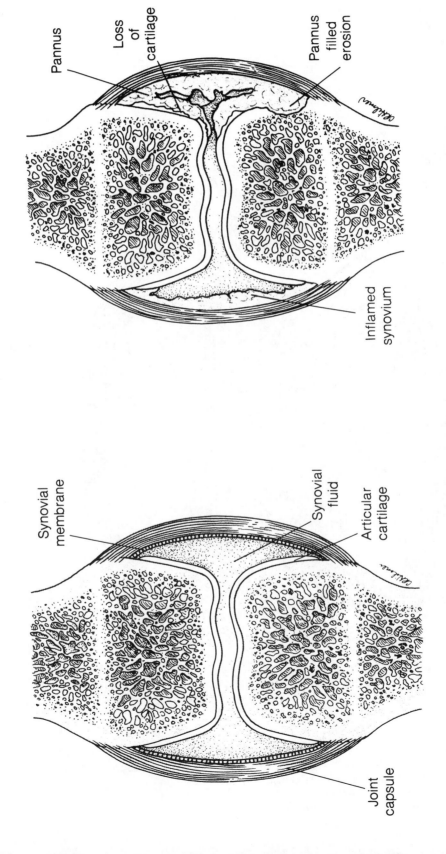

FIG. 58–1. (Left) Normal joint structures. (Right) Joint changes in rheumatoid arthritis. The left side denotes early changes occurring within the synovium, and the right side shows progressive disease that leads to erosion and the formation of pannus
Porth: Pathophysiology, 4th Edition
Copyright © 1994, J.B. Lippincott Company

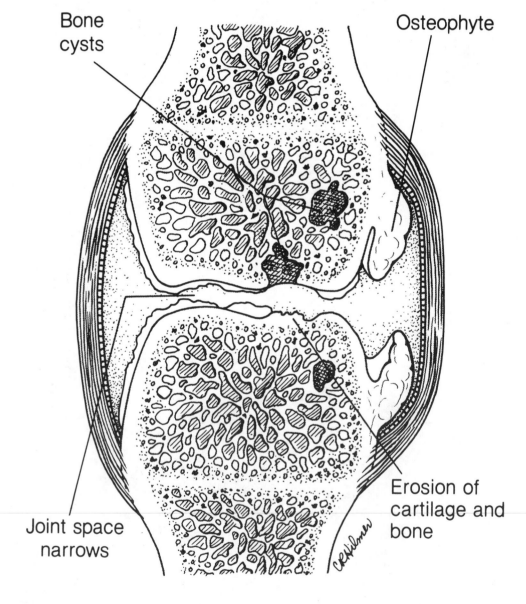

Bone
cysts

Osteophyte

Joint space
narrows

Erosion of
cartilage and
bone

FIG. 58–5. Joint changes in osteoarthritis. The left side denotes early changes and joint space narrowing with cartilage breakdown. The right side shows more severe disease progression with lost cartilage and osteophyte formation
Porth: Pathophysiology, 4th Edition
Copyright © 1994, J.B. Lippincott Company